Y0-DKY-913

ATLAS OF CANINE AND FELINE DERMATOSES

by

Robert M. Schwartzman, V.M.D., Ph.D.

*Associate Professor of Dermatology,
School of Veterinary Medicine,
University of Pennsylvania, Philadelphia*

and

Frank Král, V.M.D., Doc. habil.

*Emeritus Professor of Dermatology,
School of Veterinary Medicine,
University of Pennsylvania, Philadelphia*

302 Illustrations in Color

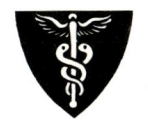

LEA & FEBIGER   1967   **PHILADELPHIA**

Copyright © November 1967 by Lea & Febiger
All Rights Reserved

Library of Congress Catalog Card Number 66-29360
Printed in the United States of America

To my Wife and Children.
                        R.M.S.

To my Parents.
                F. K.

PREFACE

Rational therapy of skin diseases requires an accurate diagnosis. The gross skin changes in the animal patient appear like an artistic picture that is produced by the skin in response to a variety of insults. The size, shape, color and type of lesion differ with the particular disease as the artistic picture varies according to the individuality of the artist. In general, a particular cause "paints" the same type of dermatologic illustration. The visual findings in the practice of dermatology are generally the primary basis for making a diagnosis. For this reason, this atlas is intended to "describe" pictorially the dermatoses commonly seen by the veterinarian in his small animal practice. The brevity of the text underscores our opinion that more can be learned by seeing a skin lesion than by reading about it. The presentation of the spectrum of lesions and the histopathologic changes associated with a particular skin disorder are intended to aid the veterinarian in his diagnosis of dermatoses. The etiology, pathogenesis and treatment are not considered because these subjects can be found in any number of veterinary textbooks.

The atlas does not claim to be complete, since it is obvious that the material presented is limited by the experience of the authors, particularly geographic. An atlas which contains the totality of animal dermatoses will be forthcoming when our experience broadens and when a larger group of veterinary dermatologists are trained and contribute to the literature. We hope that our effort will stimulate students, practitioners and scientists to engage in the rewarding investigation of veterinary dermatology not only for its own worth, i.e., the caring for animal patients, but also for yielding useful information which might serve human medicine.

Particular acknowledgment and appreciation are given to Dr. H. Beerman for his valuable advice in the preparation of the atlas; to Dr. J. Conroy, Dr. R. Kirk, Dr. G. Muller and Dr. J. Skelley for their kindness in allowing use of their pictures; and to Charles C. Thomas, Publisher, for their permission to reproduce 22 illustrations that appeared in black and white in Schwartzman, R. M. and Orkin, M.: *A Comparative Study of Skin Diseases of Dog and Man.*

Philadelphia

ROBERT M. SCHWARTZMAN
FRANK KRÁL

CONTENTS

CHAPTER 1
DEFINITIONS AND BASIC REACTIONS OF THE SKIN
Erythema	11
Macule	11
Vesicle and Bulla (Blister)	12
Exudation	12
Pustule	13
Papule, Plaque, Nodule and Tumor	13
Wheal	14
Lichenification	15
Vitiligo (Depigmentation)	15
Comedo	15
Alopecia	16
Necrosis	16
Scale	17
Crust	17
Ulcer	18
Histology and Histopathologic Reactions	18

CHAPTER 2
ALLERGIC DERMATOSES
Urticaria	28
Pollinosis (Atopy)	30
Allergic Contact Dermatitis	31
Solar Dermatitis	32
Arthropod Reactions	34

CHAPTER 3
PYODERMA—(Bacterial Infection of the Skin)
Impetigo	39
Folliculitis (superficial)	40
Furunculosis	41
Hidradenitis suppurativa	44

Juvenile Pyoderma ... 45
Necrotizing Pyoderma ... 45
Bacterial Paronychia ... 46
Secondary Pyoderma ... 46

Chapter 4
SPECIFIC INFECTIONS WITH CUTANEOUS MANIFESTATIONS
Leptospirosis ... 51
Hard Pad Disease ... 51
North American Blastomycosis ... 51
Nocardiosis ... 52

Chapter 5
SCABIES ... 53

Chapter 6
DEMODECTIC MANGE
Localized ... 55
Generalized ... 56

Chapter 7
RHABDITIC DERMATITIS ... 59

Chapter 8
CHEYLETIELLA PARASITIVORAX DERMATITIS ... 61

Chapter 9
NOTOEDRIC MANGE ... 63

Chapter 10
DERMATOMYCOSIS ... 64

Chapter 11
MONILIASIS ... 68

CHAPTER 12
SEBORRHEA   70

CHAPTER 13
FACIAL KERATOSIS AND FOLLICULAR KERATOSIS   73

CHAPTER 14
THALLIUM INTOXICATION   74

CHAPTER 15
CALLUS   77

CHAPTER 16
ACRAL-PRURITIC NODULE   79

CHAPTER 17
SLOUGH   81

CHAPTER 18
INTERTRIGO   82
Perivulvar Intertrigo   82
Lip Fold Pyoderma   82

CHAPTER 19
EOSINOPHILIC GRANULOMA   83

CHAPTER 20
LINEAR GRANULOMA   83

CHAPTER 21
ACNE   86

CHAPTER 22
HORMONAL DERMATOSES
Hypothyroidism   88
Acanthosis Nigricans   90
Gonadal-adrenal Dysfunction   92
Testicular Dysfunction   92

Hypoandrogenism	94
Ovarian Dysfunction	95
Changes Occurring with Castration	99
Adrenal Dysfunction	100
Cutaneous Lesion Associated with Increased 17-Ketosteroid Output	105

INDEX	110

CHAPTER
1
DEFINITIONS and BASIC REACTIONS of SKIN

Erythema.

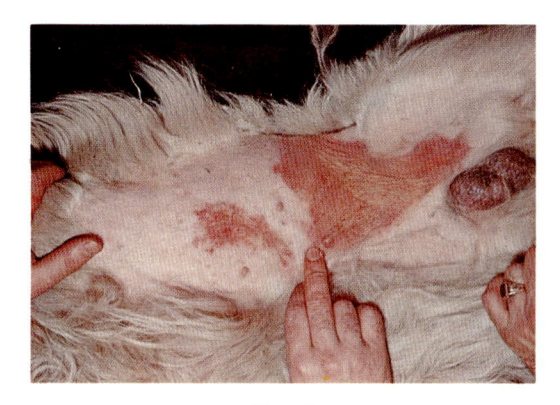

Fig. 1
Reddening of the skin.

Macule. Non-elevated lesion in which there is a change in the color of the skin.

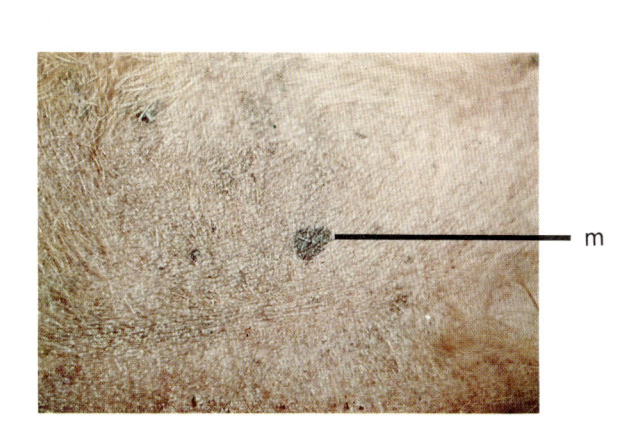

Fig. 2
Hyperpigmented macule (m) as occurs in a nevus.

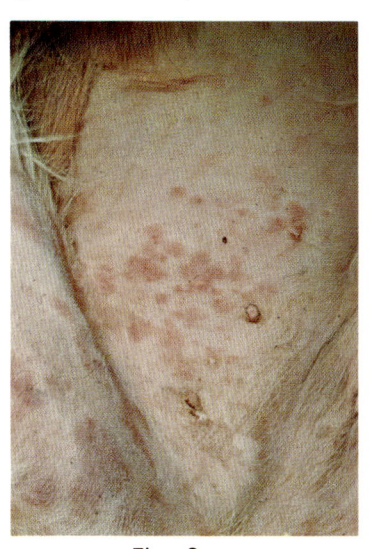

Fig. 3
Erythematous macules.

Vesicle and Bulla (blister). Sharply circumscribed collections of serous fluid on the skin producing an elevated lesion. A vesicle is less than 1 cm. in diameter and a bulla greater than 1 cm.

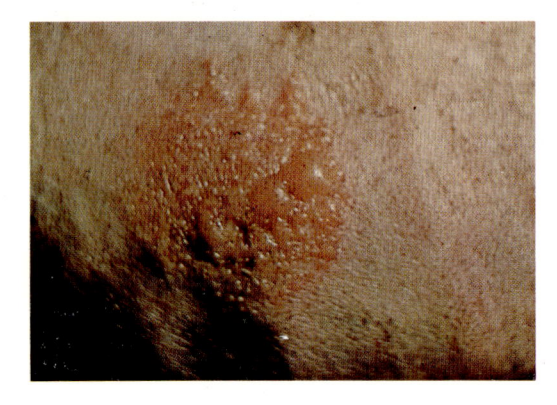

Fig. 4

Exudation. The transit of tissue fluid through the epidermis (more common than vesiculation in animal skin).

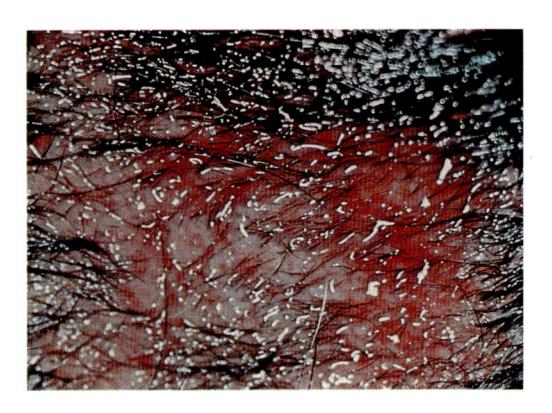

Fig. 5 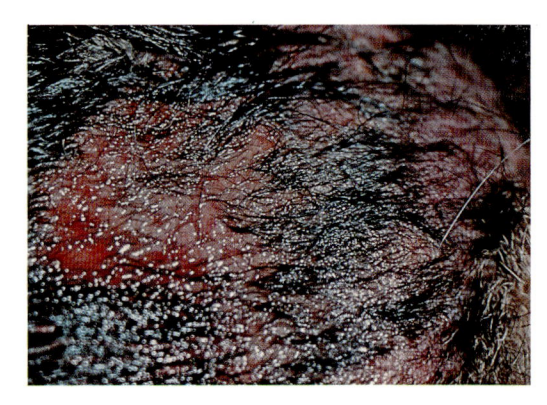   Fig. 6

Pustule. A circumscribed collection of purulent material on the skin.

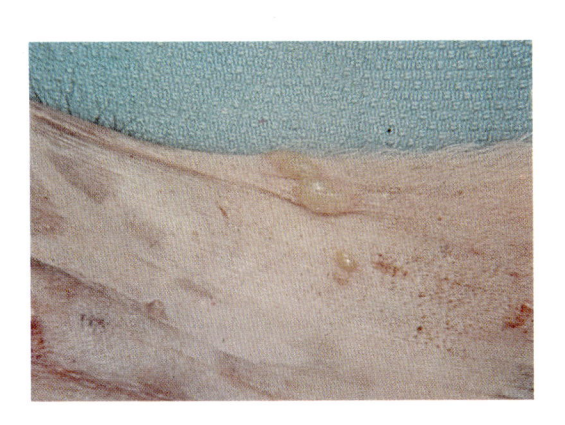

Fig. 7

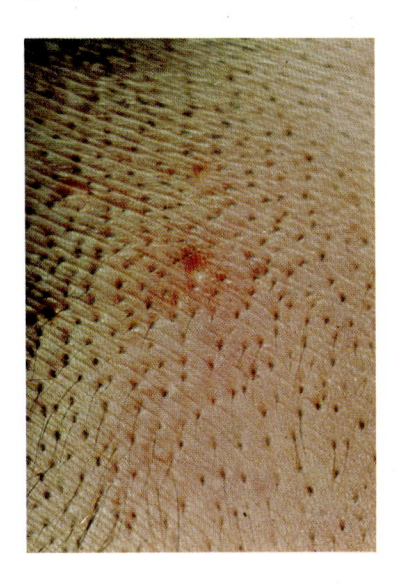

Fig. 8

Papule, Plaque, Nodule, and Tumor. Solid elevated lesions on the skin. Papules are less than 1 cm. in size; plaques are larger infiltrated areas; and nodules and tumors are deeper and larger solitary lesions of the skin and subcutis.

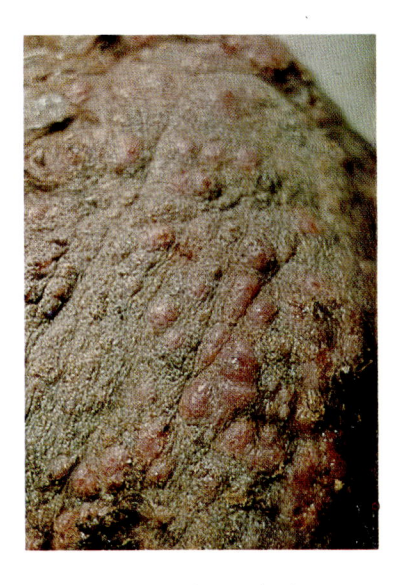

Fig. 9 (Papules)

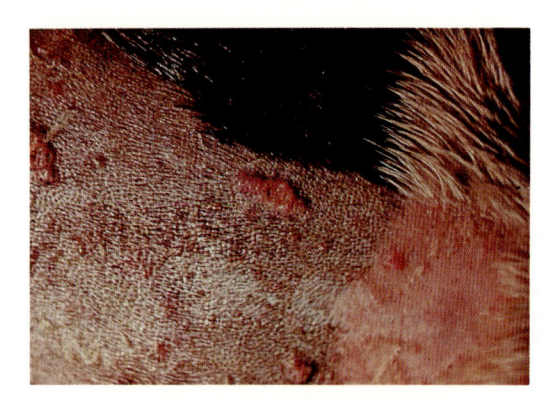

Fig. 10 (Plaque)

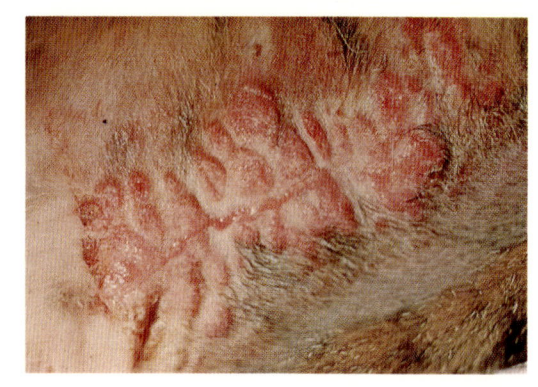

Fig. 11 (Plaque)

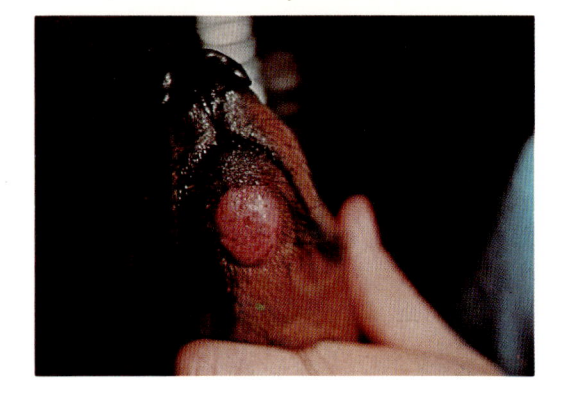

Fig. 12 (Nodule)

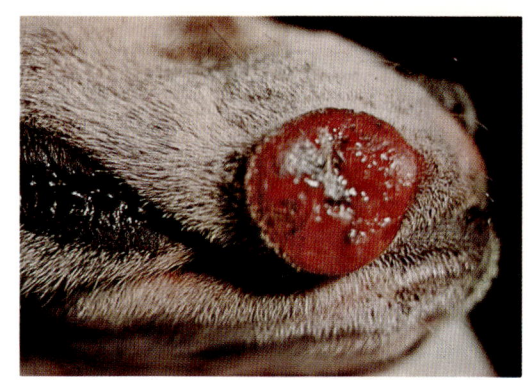

Fig. 13 (Tumor)

Wheal. A sharply circumscribed steep-walled and flat-topped elevation of the skin resulting from a histamine reaction in the dermis.

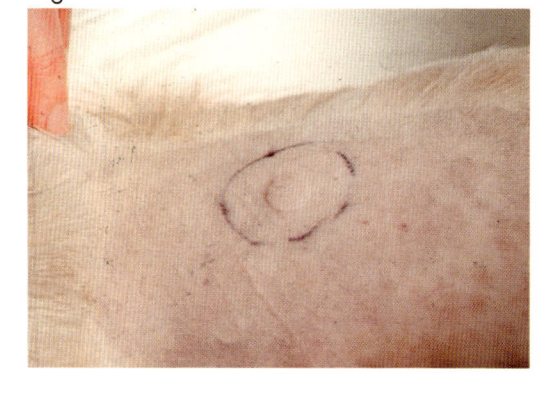

Fig. 14

Lichenification. A form of chronic dermatitis in which the skin markings are accentuated, resulting in a bark-like appearance of the skin. Hyperpigmentation often is associated.

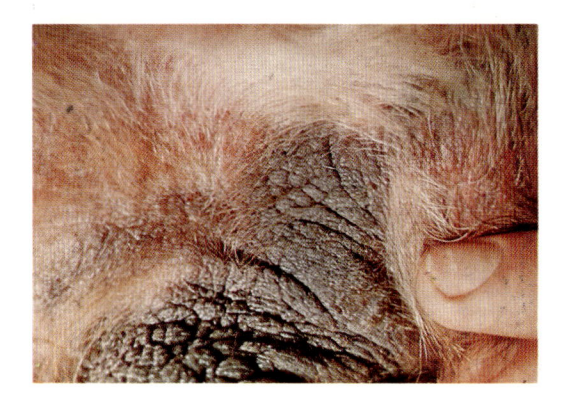

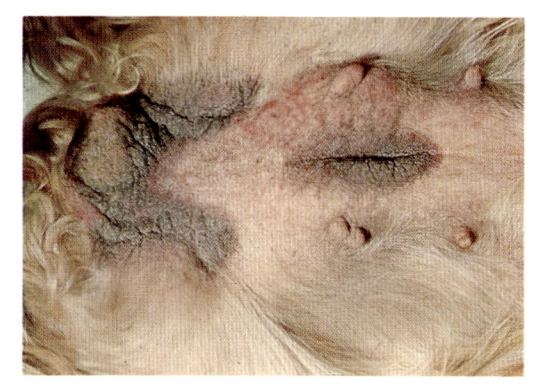

Fig. 15

Fig. 16

Vitiligo (depigmentation). White patches of the skin due to loss of pigment without other trophic changes.

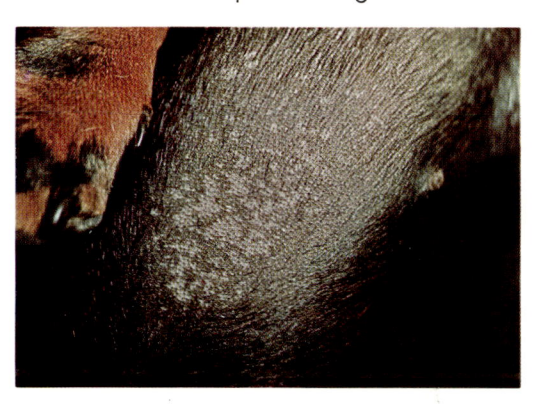

Fig. 17

Comedo (c) (pl., comedones). A plug of sebaceous material capped with a blackened mass, filling the pilosebaceous orifice.

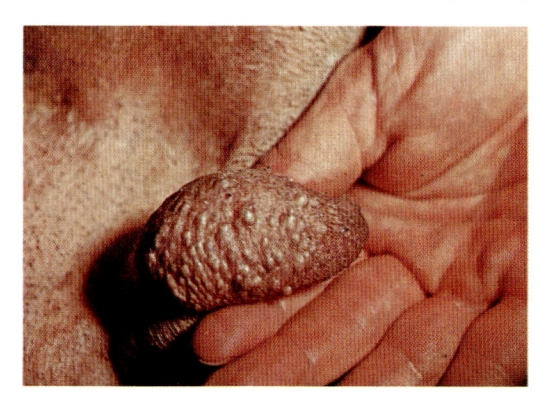

Fig. 18

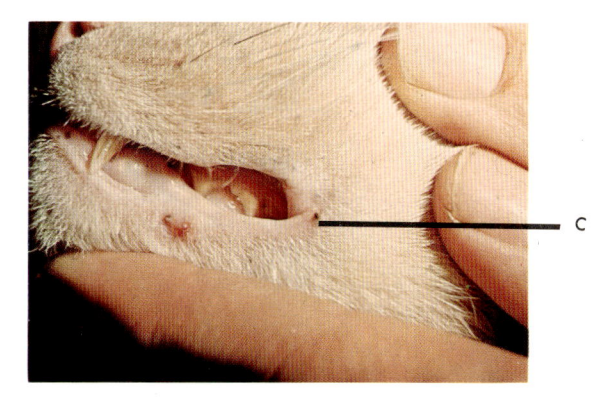

Fig. 19

Alopecia. The loss of hair.

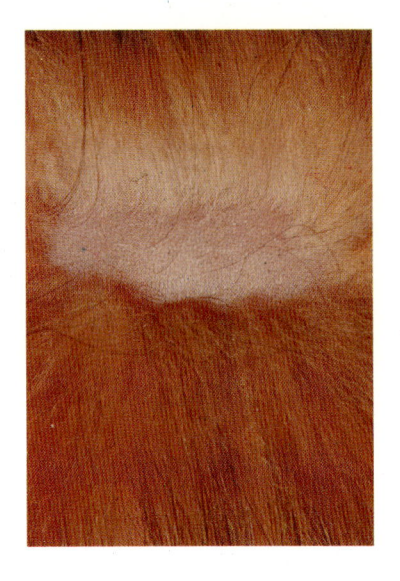

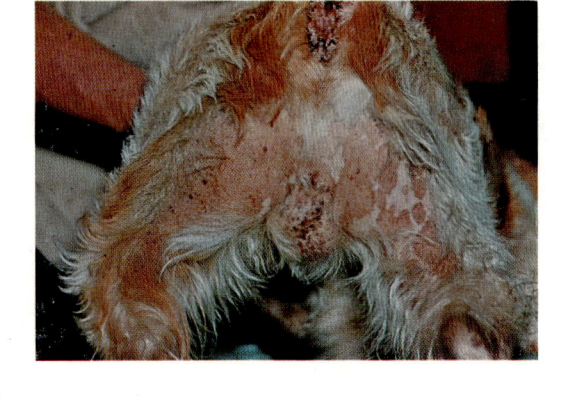

Fig. 21

Fig. 20

Necrosis. Death of one or more cells or of a portion of tissue or organ.

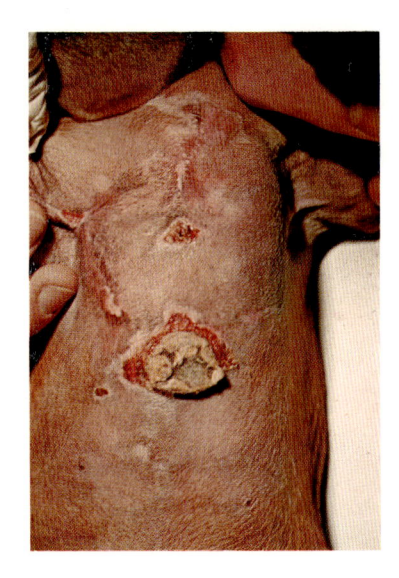

Fig. 22

Scale. Accumulation of loose, horny fragments of the stratum corneum.

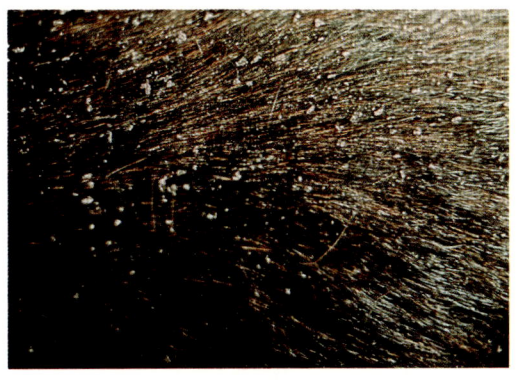

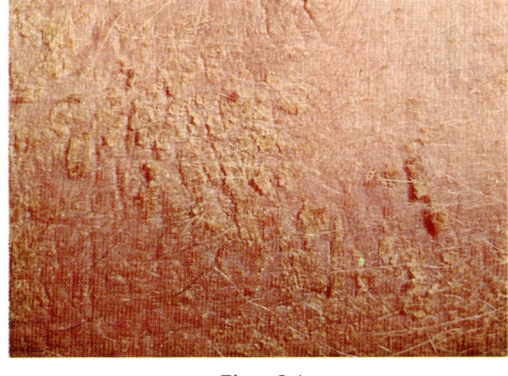

Fig. 23

Fig. 24

Crust. Dried remains of exudate from erosive, exudative or ulcerated lesion.

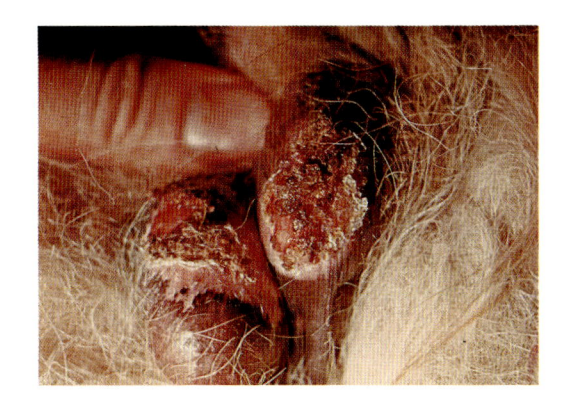

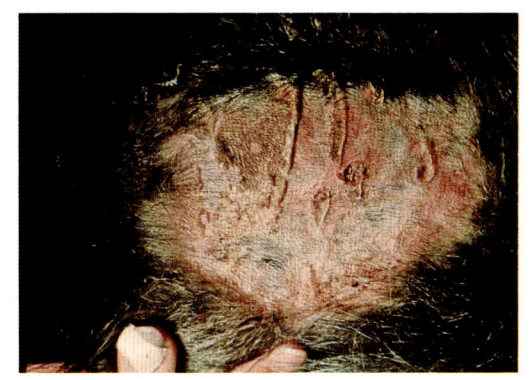

Fig. 25

Fig. 26

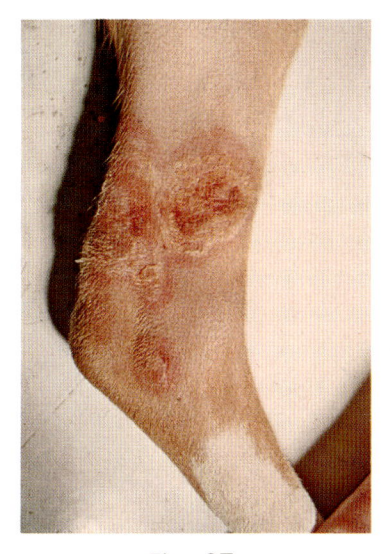

Fig. 27

Ulcer. Loss of continuity of skin surface caused by a destructive process which removes the epidermis and extends into the dermis.

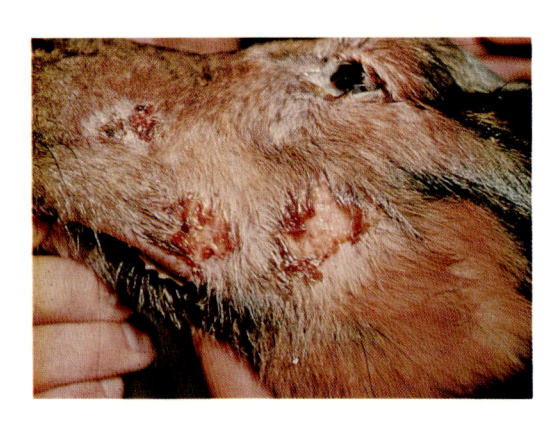

Fig. 28

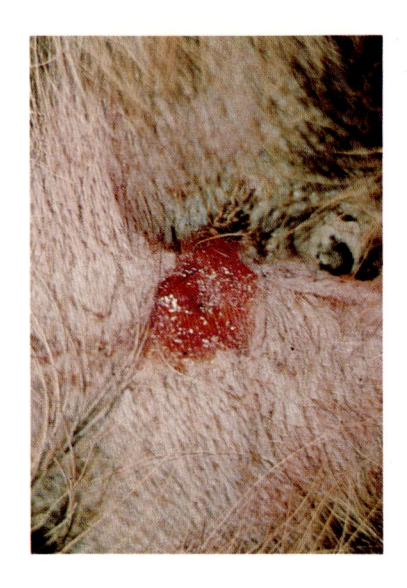

Fig. 29

HISTOLOGY and HISTOPATHOLOGIC REACTIONS

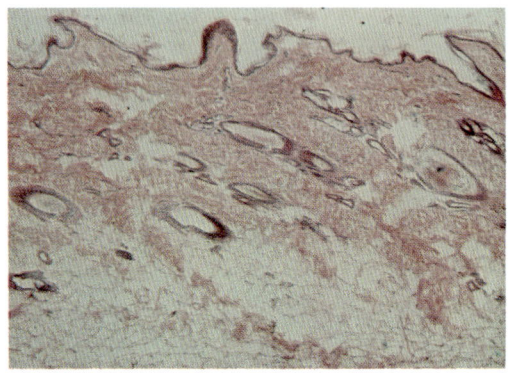

Fig. 30

Skin of normal dog. Note undulating surface, thinness of epidermis and abundance of appendages. H. & E., × 35.

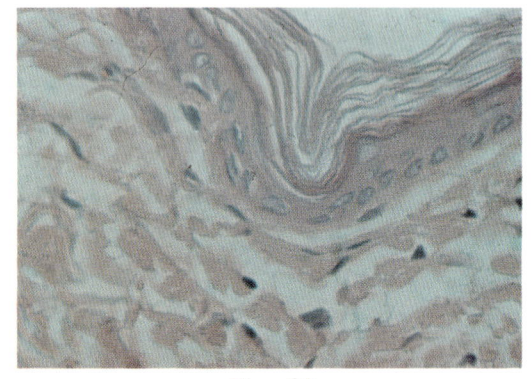

Fig. 31

Epidermis of normal dog. Note thinness of epidermis—absence of rete ridges and granular cell layer. H. & E., × 450.

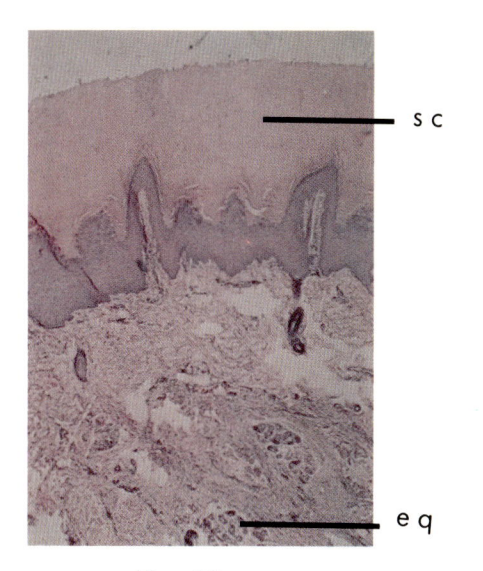

Fig. 32

Pad of normal dog. Note massive stratum corneum (s c), highly developed prickle-cell layer, and eccrine sweat glands (e g). H. & E., × 35.

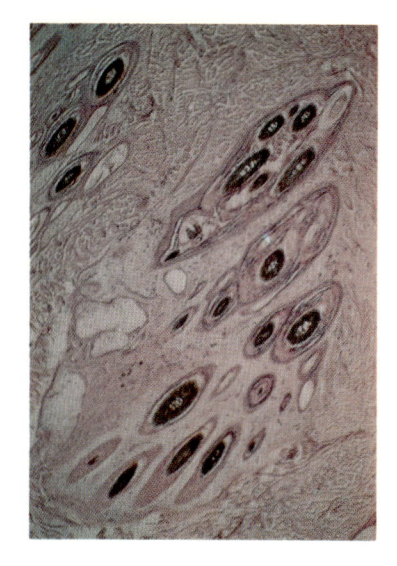

Fig. 33

Skin of normal dog. Note uppermost follicle containing multiple hairs which results from convergence of accessory follicles into a primary follicle in the upper one-third of the dermis. H. & E., × 35.

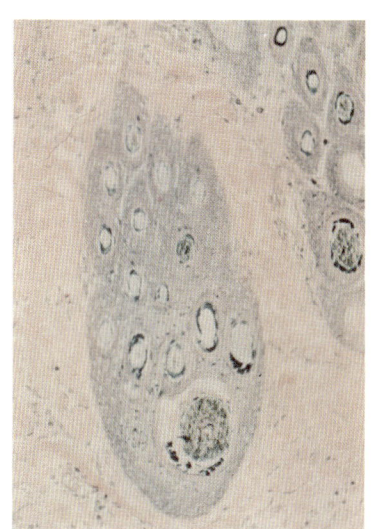

Fig. 34

Skin of normal dog. Note grouping of primary and accessory follicles in lower part of the dermis. H. & E., × 100.

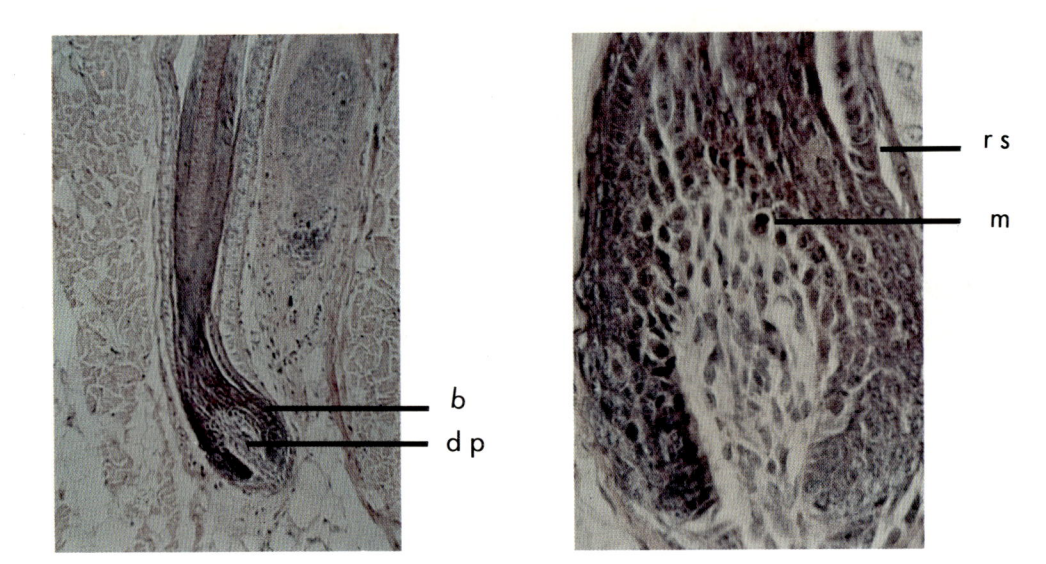

Figs. 35 and 36

Anagen (growing) hair follicle* (in longitudinal section) of normal canine skin. Note dermal papilla (d p), bulb (b), melanocytes (m) and root sheaths (r s). H. & E., × 35 and × 450.

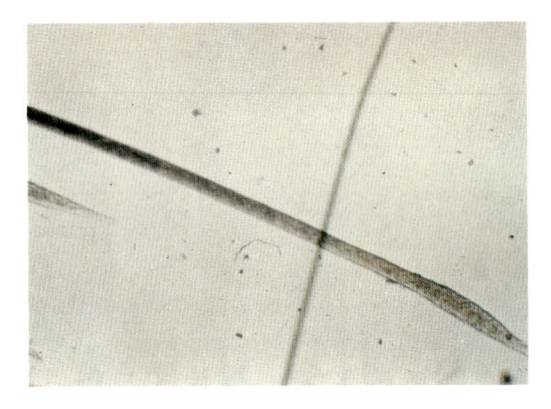

Fig. 37

Telogen (resting) dog hair (plucked). Note pointed appearance of hair tip, absence of root sheaths and paucity of pigment. × 100.

*The hair follicle goes through alternate periods of activity (anagen) and resting (telogen). An intermediate stage is referred to as catagen.

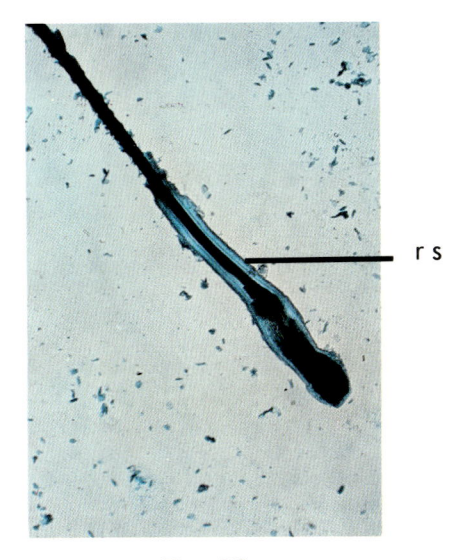

Fig. 38
Anagen dog hair (plucked). Note darkly pigmented bulbous tip and extensive root sheaths (r s). Lacto phenol cotton blue × 100.

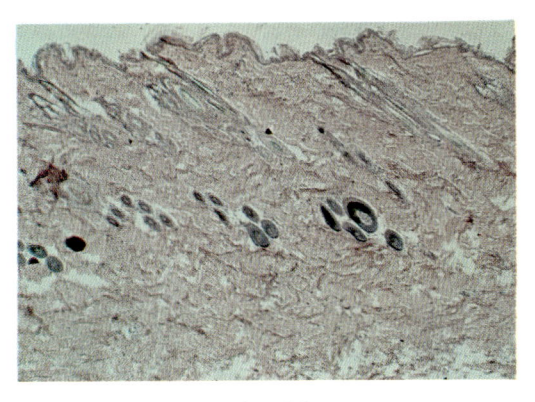

Fig. 39
Skin of normal cat. Note undulating surface, thin epidermis and abundance of appendages. H. & E., × 35.

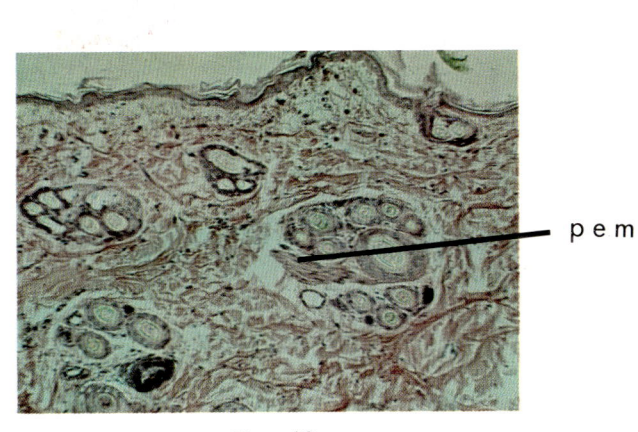

Fig. 40
Skin of normal cat. Note thin epidermis, pilo-erector muscle (p e m) and aggregations of primary and accessory follicles. H. & E., × 100.

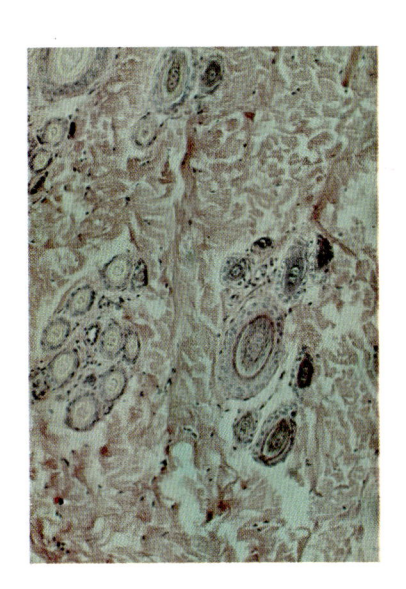

Fig. 41
Skin of normal cat. Note grouping of follicles deep in dermis. H. & E., × 100.

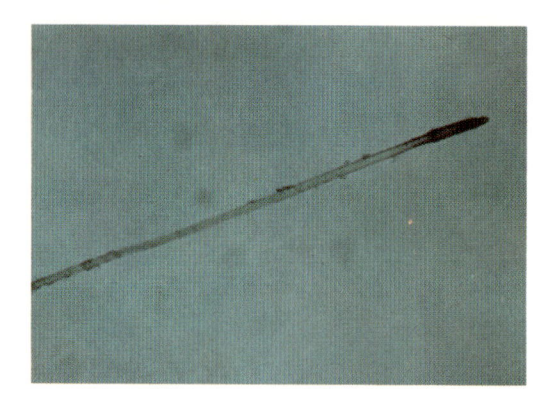

Fig. 42
Telogen cat hair (plucked). Note pointed appearance of hair tip, absence of root sheaths and paucity of pigment. × 35.

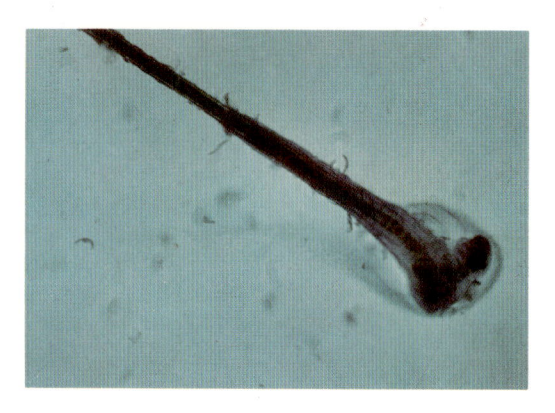

Fig. 43
Anagen cat hair (plucked). Note darkly pigmented bulbous tip. Lacto phenol cotton blue × 100.

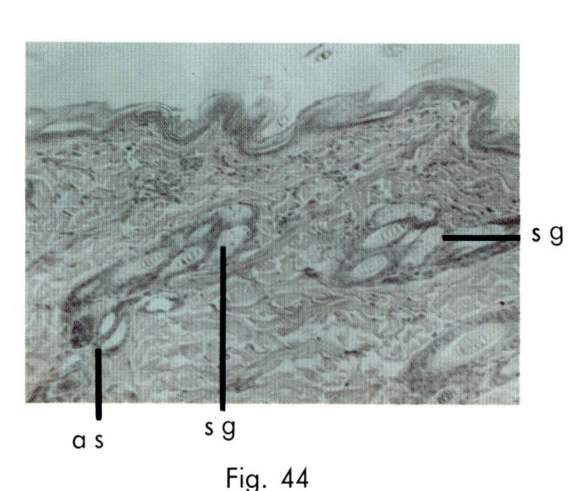

Fig. 44
Skin of normal cat. Note sebaceous glands (s g) and apocrine structures (a s). H. & E., × 100.

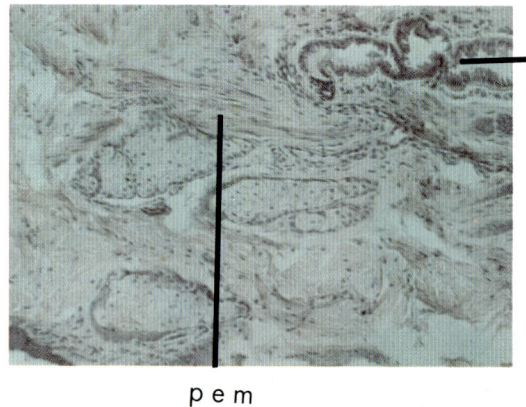

Fig. 45
Skin of normal dog. Note apocrine structures (a s) and pilo-erector muscle (p e m). H. & E., × 100.

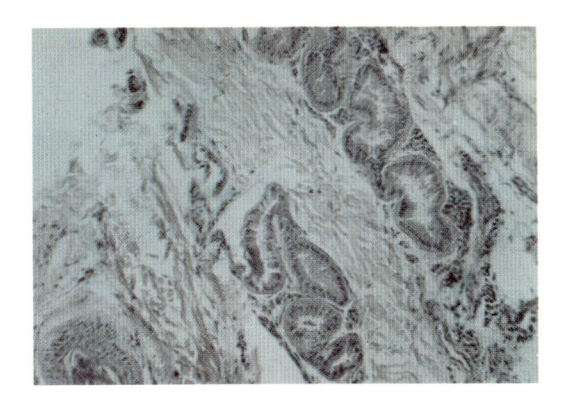

Fig. 46

Skin of normal dog. Note apocrine structures deep in dermis. H. & E., × 100.

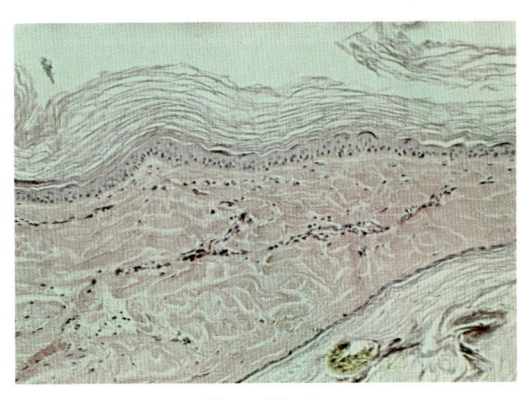

Fig. 47 A 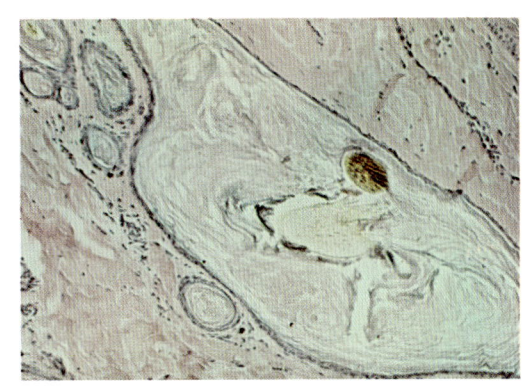   Fig. 47 B

Hyperkeratosis. An increased thickness in the stratum corneum. On surface epidermis (A) and in follicle (B). Hypothyroidism (canine). H. & E., × 100.

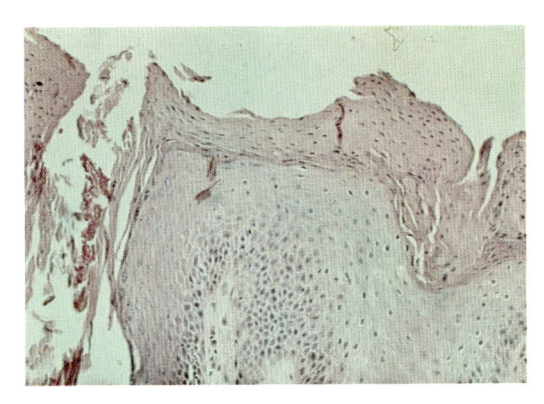

Fig. 48 A 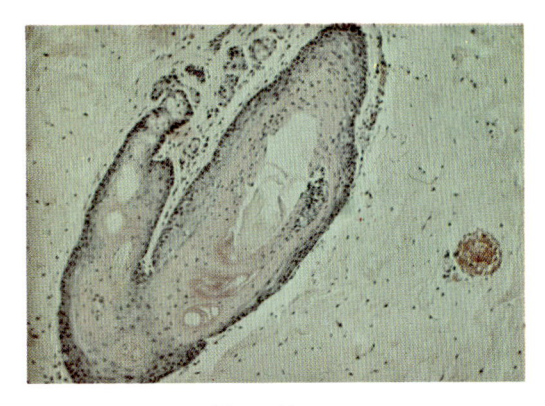   Fig. 48 B

Parakeratosis. The presence of nucleated cells in the stratum corneum. Thallium intoxication (canine). H. & E., × 100.

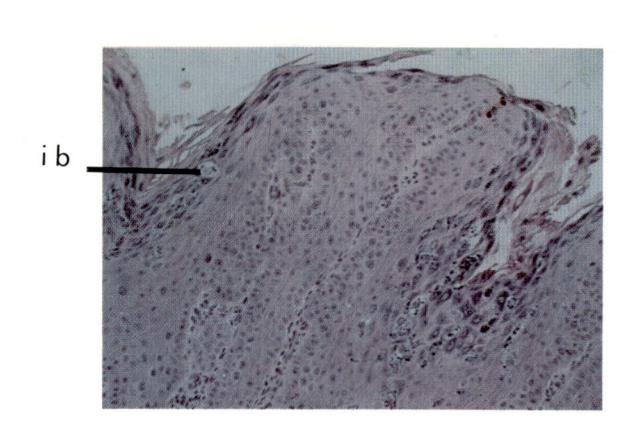

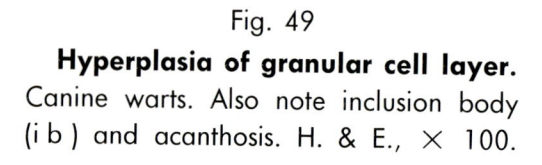

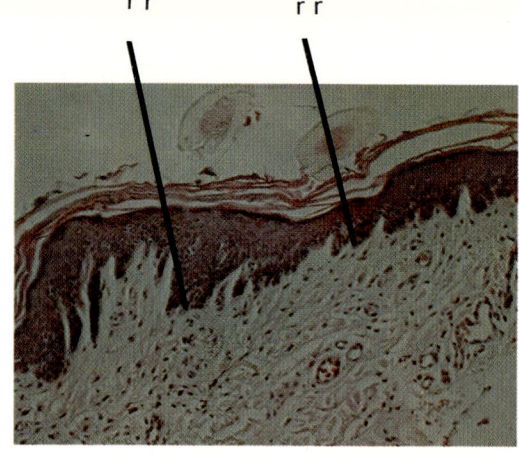

Fig. 49
Hyperplasia of granular cell layer. Canine warts. Also note inclusion body (i b) and acanthosis. H. & E., × 100.

Fig. 50
Acanthosis. Hyperplasia of the Malpighian layer—also note development of rete ridges (r r). H. & E., × 100.

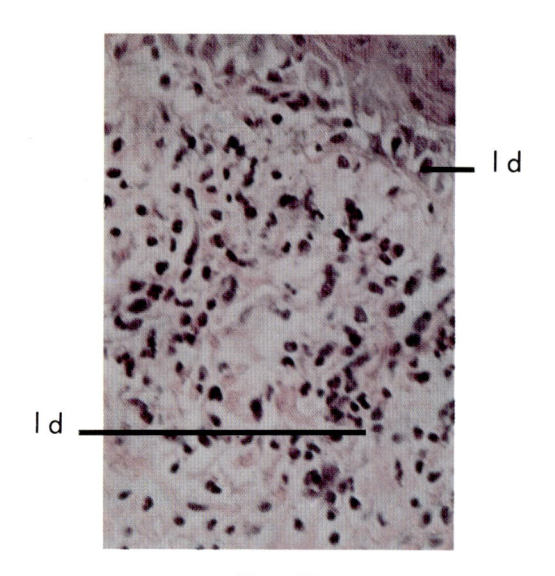

Fig. 51

Liquefaction degeneration (l.d.) of basal layer. A type of hydropic degeneration causing disintegration and vacuolization of basal cells. Insect bite (canine). H. & E., × 100.

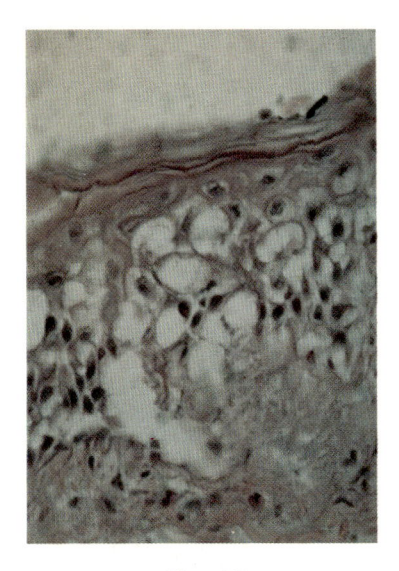

Fig. 52

Reticular degeneration. Severe intracellular edema causes bursting of epidermal cells and the formation of multilocular bullae. Urticaria (canine). H. & E., × 450.

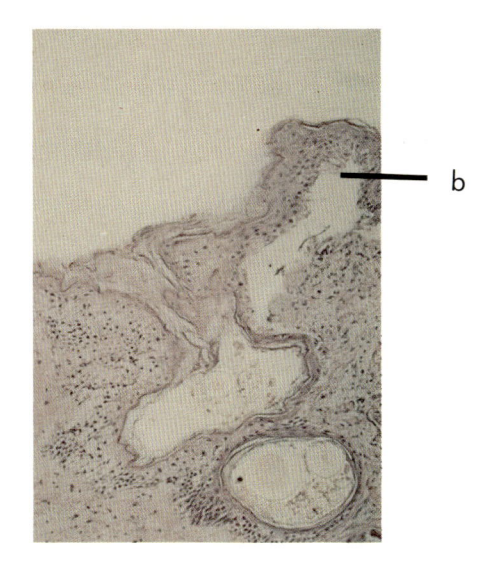

Fig. 53

Bulla (b). A cavity within or under the epidermis filled with tissue fluid. Urticaria (canine). H. & E., × 100. (Also see Fig. 61.)

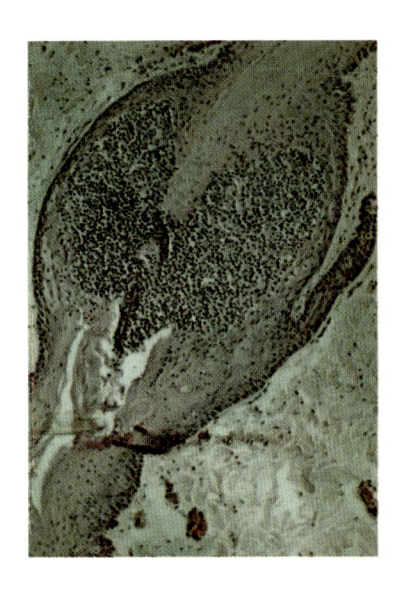

Fig. 54

Spongiform pustule. A multilocular pustule in which neutrophils appear inside edematous epidermal cells and a spongelike network is formed by the cellular wall remnants of ruptured cells. Thallium intoxication (dog-hair follicle). H. & E., × 100.

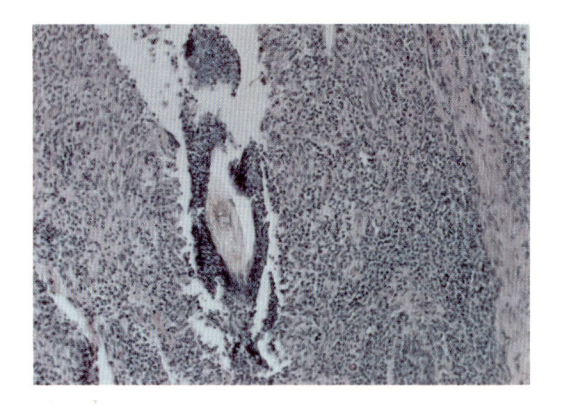

Fig. 55
Follicular destruction. The loss of the follicular appendage as a result of the invasion of inflammatory cells. Ringworm (canine). H. & E., × 100.

Fig. 56 A

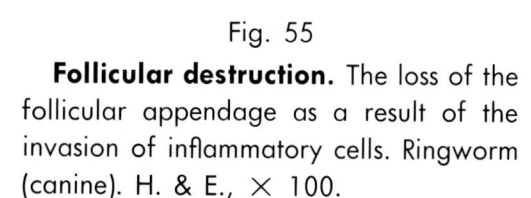

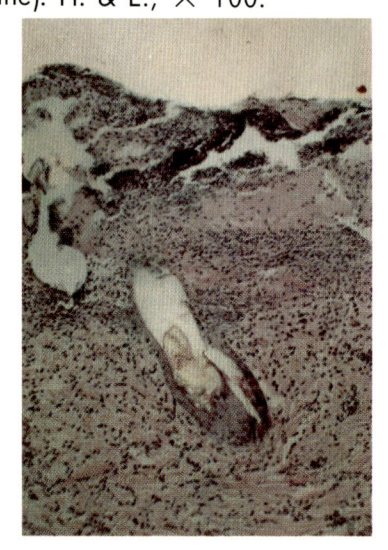

Fig. 56 B

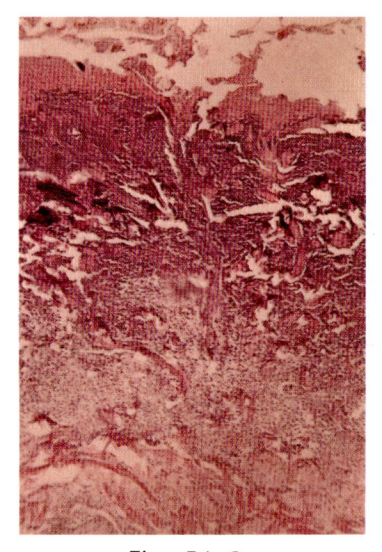

Fig. 56 C

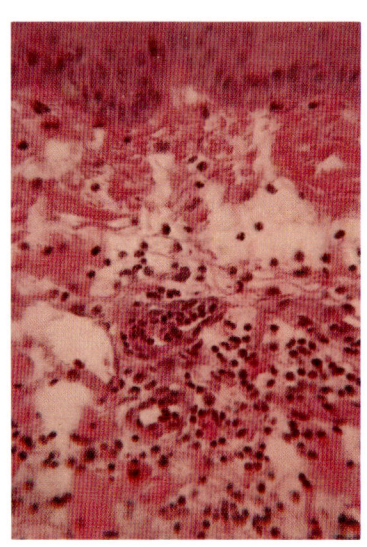

Fig. 56 D

Acute dermatitis. The usual findings are that the epidermis is absent and replaced by an inflammatory crust. In the upper one-third of the dermis are acute inflammatory changes (edema, neutrophils, etc.). H. & E., × 35, 35, 100 and 450.

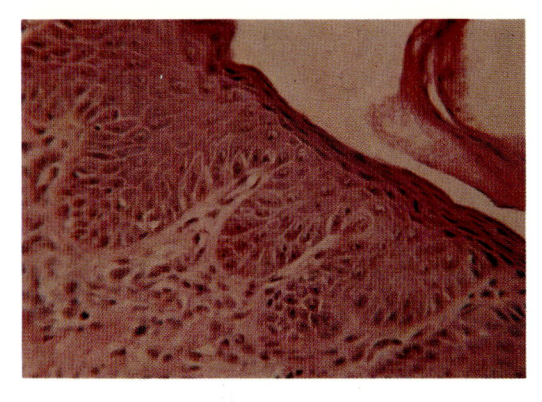

Fig. 57 A

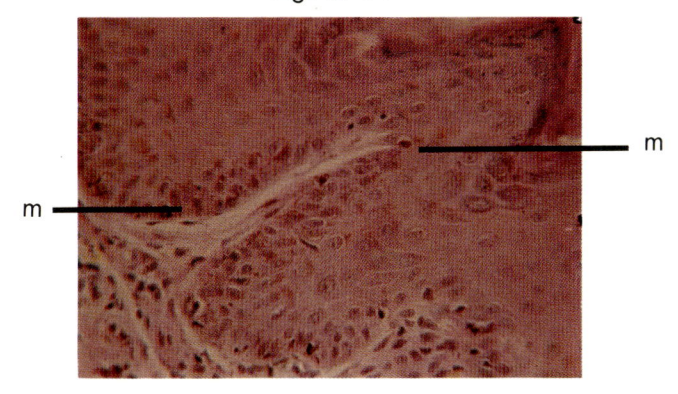

Fig. 57 B

Chronic dermatitis. The epidermal changes are hyperkeratosis or parakeratosis, acanthosis and an increase in melanin (m) production. The dermal pattern is variable, but mononuclear cells rather than neutrophils occur in the inflammatory infiltrate. H. & E., × 450.

CHAPTER
2

ALLERGIC DERMATOSES
A. URTICARIA

An immediate type of hypersensitivity resulting in the release of histamine and the formation of hives (wheals). Causative may be allergic digestants, contactants or inhalants. Pruritus may or may not be present.

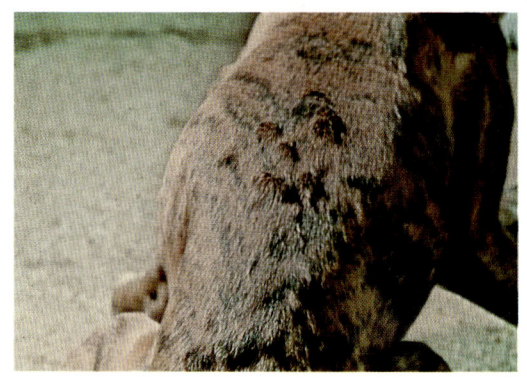

Fig. 58

The lesions occur primarily on the trunk and appear as "bumps" or nodules in the skin. The overlying hair is disheveled.

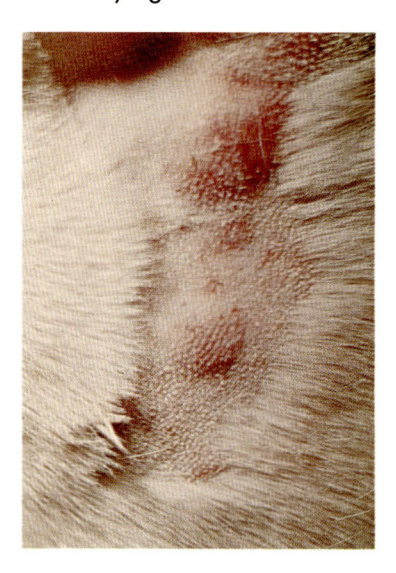

Fig. 59

When the hair is removed, a steep-walled, flat-topped nodule is evident. Varying degrees of erythema and occasionally hemorrhage are present.

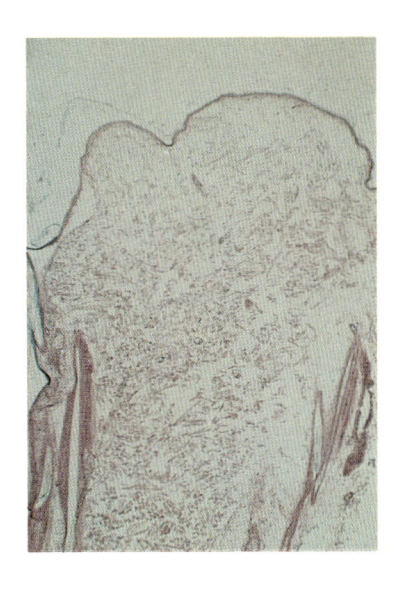

Fig. 60

The predominant reactions are massive edema and vascular dilatation. Note tearing apart of the collagen fibers. H. & E., × 35.

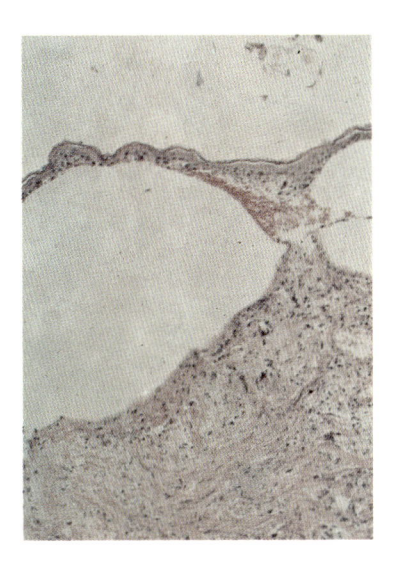

Fig. 61

Biopsy of lesion (Fig. 58). Note sub-basalar edema and hemorrhage in upper part of dermis. H. & E., × 100.

B. POLLINOSIS (ATOPY)

An immediate type of hypersensitivity characterized by pruritus—particularly facial, axillary and pedal. The disease usually is seasonal (varying with the pollen or allergen to which the animal is allergic).

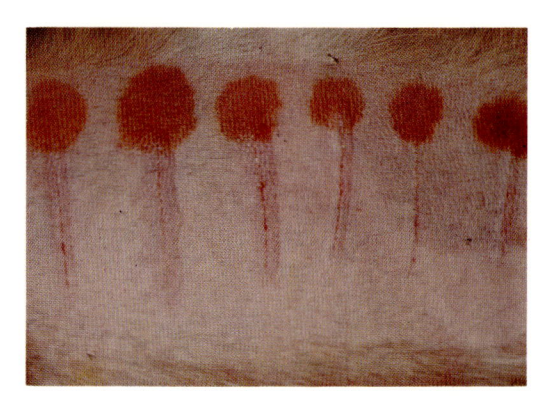

Fig. 62

Scratch test of an allergic patient. Second scratch from right is the control, fourth and fifth scratches are positive (hive) reactions to short and giant ragweed.

C. ALLERGIC CONTACT DERMATITIS

A delayed type of hypersensitivity in which an over-reactive skin responds to contact with an agent, at a non-irritating threshold. Lesions occur on hairless or relatively hairless areas (as the groin, scrotum, interdigital webs), and when induced experimentally are erythematous and papular.

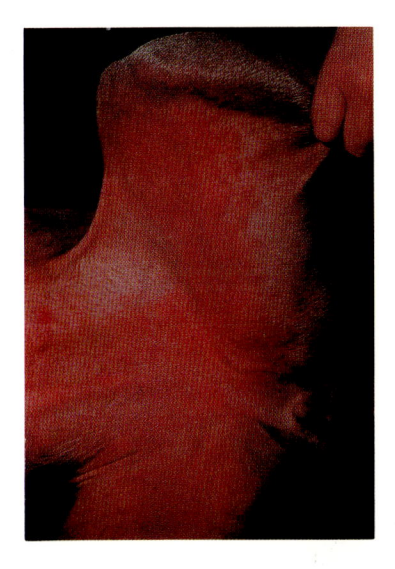

Fig. 63
A presumptive case of allergic contact dermatitis. An erythematous and papular eruption on the groin.

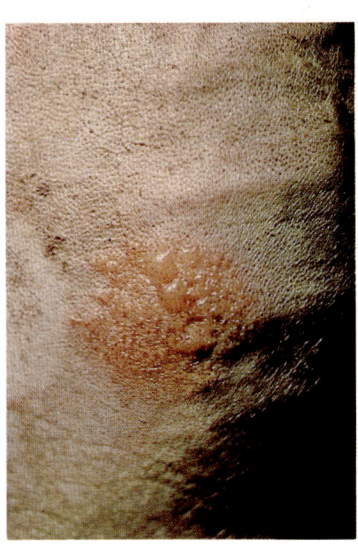

Fig. 64
Experimentally induced allergic contact dermatitis in the Mexican Hairless dog to Rhus (poison ivy). The reaction is vesicular.

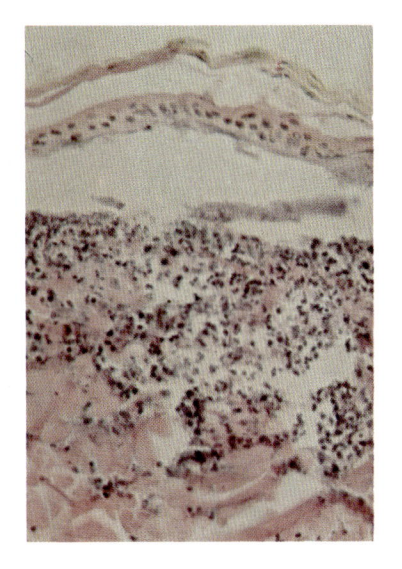

Fig. 65
Biopsy of lesion (Fig. 64). Note subbasalar edema and lymphocytic infiltrate in upper aspects of dermis. The epidermis becomes spongiotic and eventually ulcerates. H. & E., × 450.

D. SOLAR DERMATITIS

A hypersensitivity reaction to sunlight principally involving the exposed, non-haired integument: nares, eyelids and lips. Collies, Shetland Sheep dogs and related mixed breeds are particularly prone to the disease.

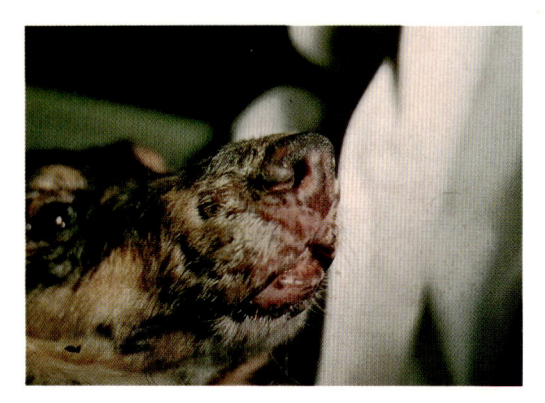

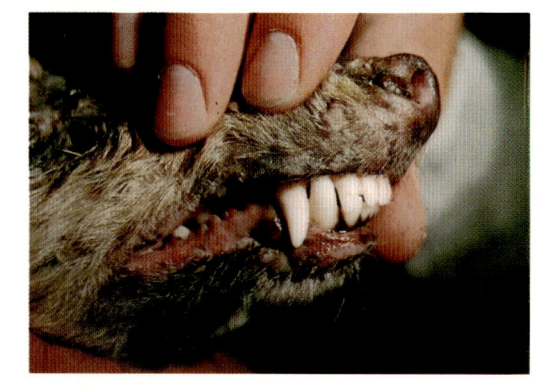

Fig. 66 A

Fig. 66 B

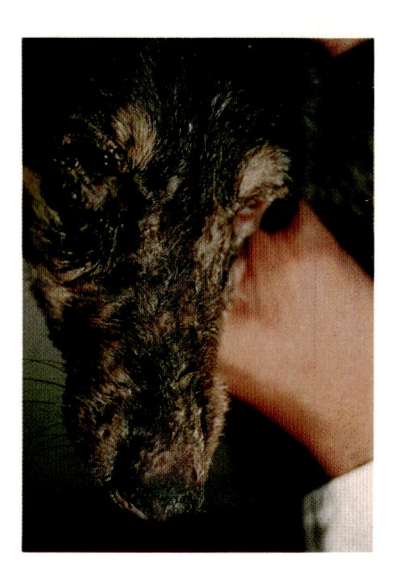

Fig. 66 C

Depigmentation of the nares, and alopecia and crusting on the peri-labial areas are characteristic. The dorsum of the nose shows alopecia and an exudative and crusting reaction.

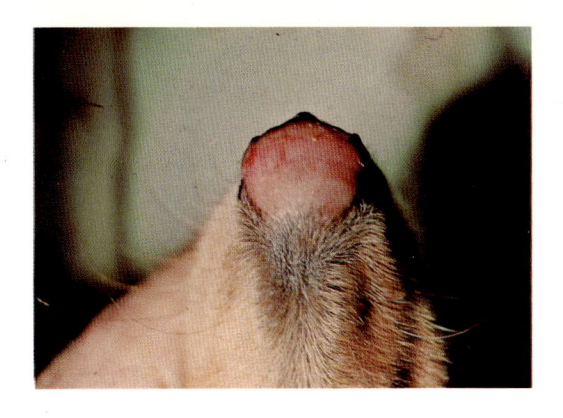

Fig. 67
Note depigmentation and erythema on dorsal aspect of muzzle.

E. ARTHROPOD REACTIONS

The lesion produced by a variety of insects often results from the salivary secretion of allergens and/or toxins. In the hypersensitive animal, intense pruritus is associated with the bite. The results of self-inflicted trauma and secondary bacterial infection often mask the primary lesion and are the presenting signs.

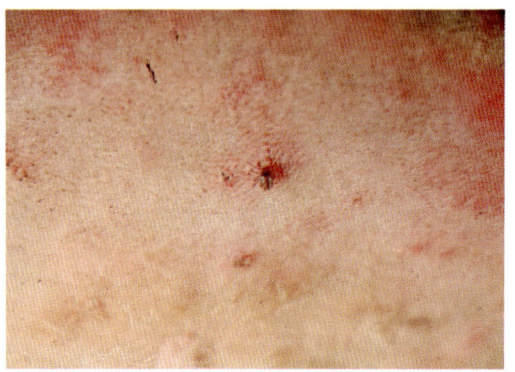

Fig. 68 A

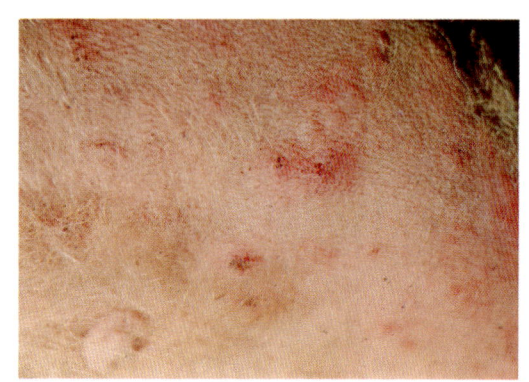

Fig. 68 B

Tick bites. Erythematous nodules with central ulceration result from the bites of ticks (A. shows tick attached to skin, and B. the resulting lesion).

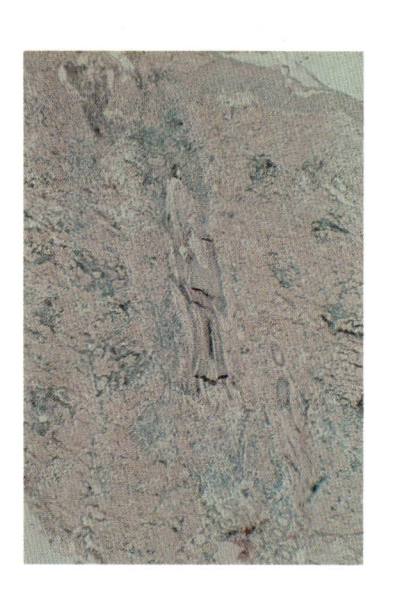

Fig. 69
Biopsy of tick bite (Fig. 68). Note acanthosis, inflammatory cell infiltration of epidermis and spotty dense inflammatory infiltrate throughout dermis. H. & E., × 35.

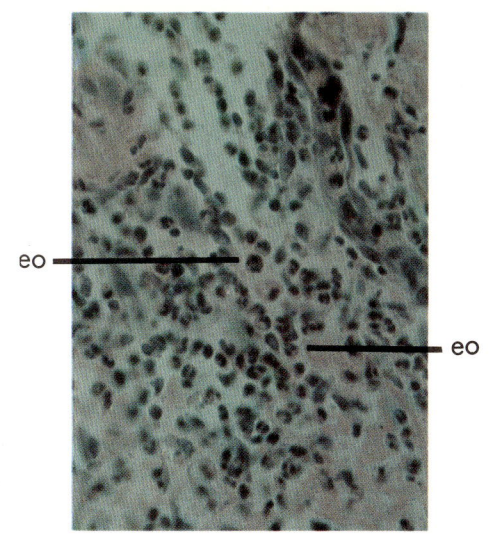

Fig. 70

Biopsy of tick bite (Fig. 68). Eosinophils (eo) and histiocytes are the predominate inflammatory cells in the dermis. H. & E., × 450.

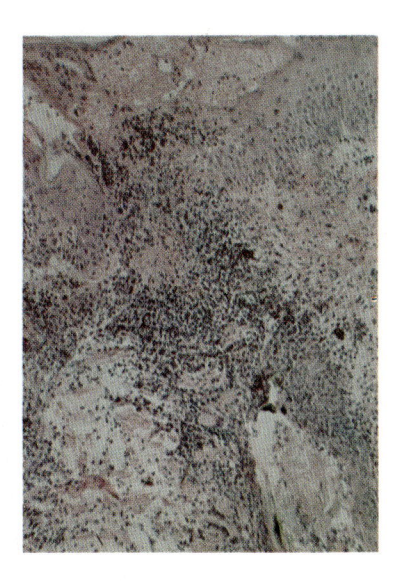

Fig. 71

Biopsy of lesion (Fig. 68). Note hemorrhage, necrosis and dense inflammatory infiltrate. H. & E., × 100.

Fig. 72 A

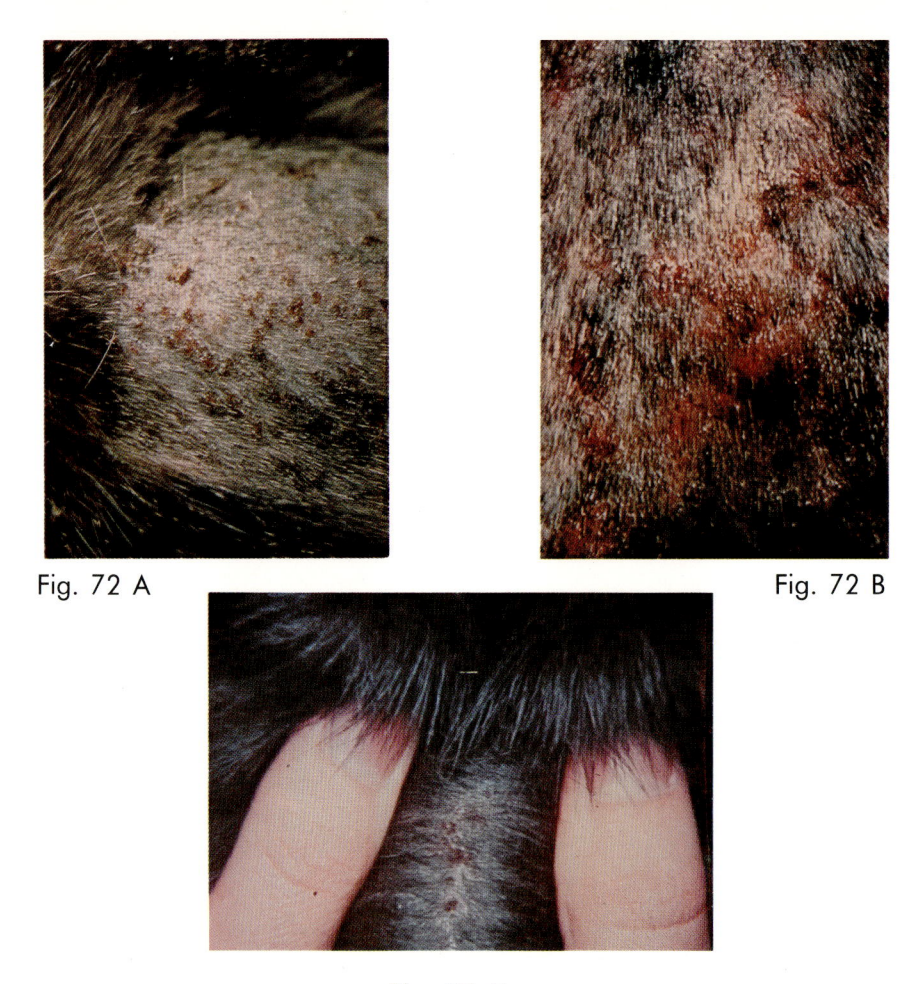

Fig. 72 B

Fig. 72 C

Flea bite (Cat)-hair has been removed for visualization of lesions. Multiple papules and erythematous crusts occur on lower parts of the back.

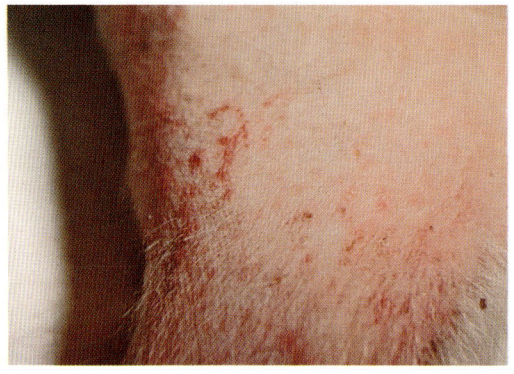

Fig. 73
Flea bites. Papular eruption on thigh.

36

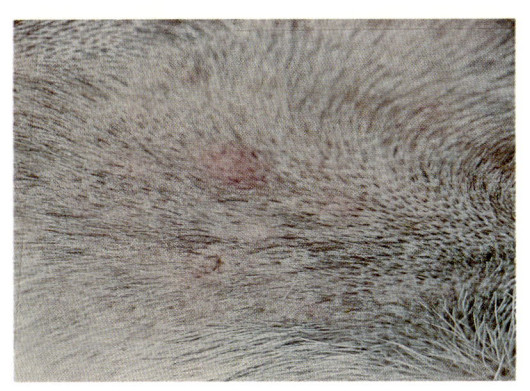

Fig. 74

Flea bites. Urticarial lesions on chest.

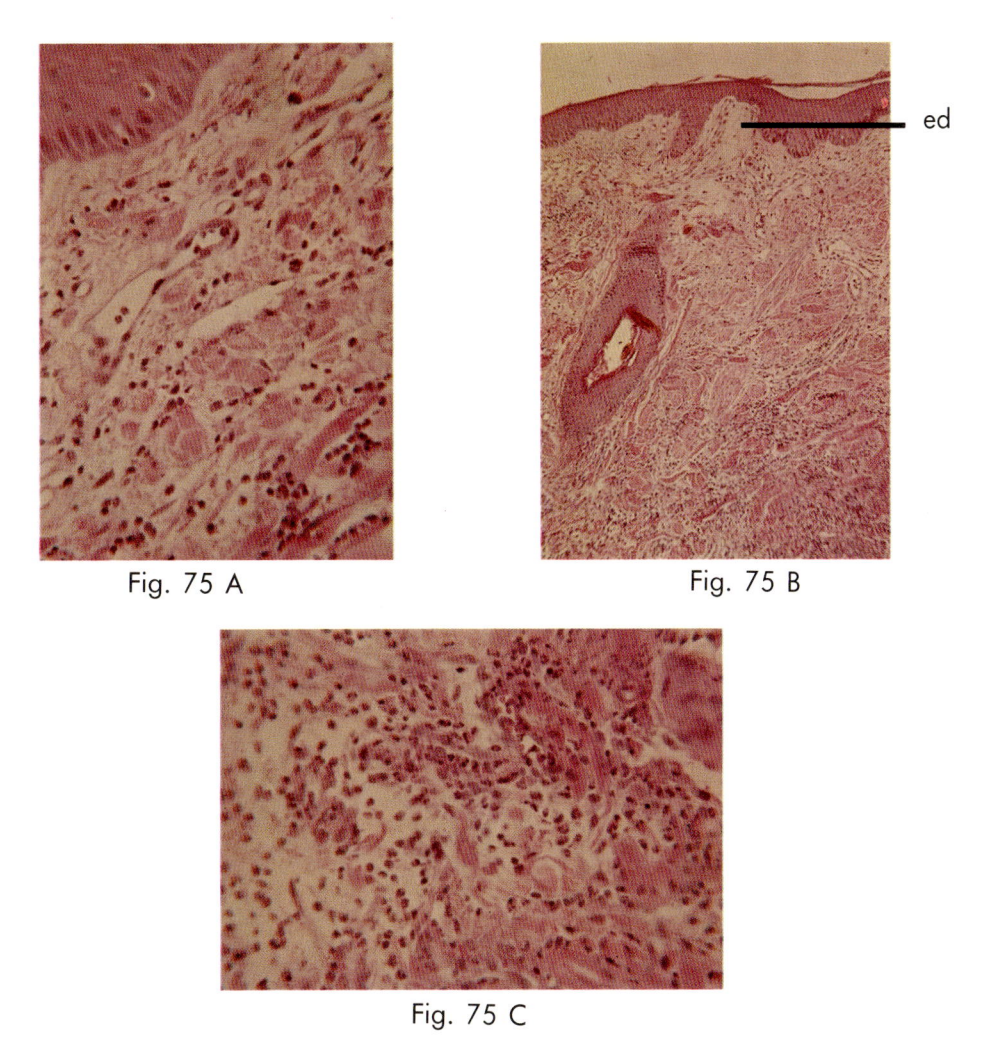

Fig. 75 A

Fig. 75 B

Fig. 75 C

Flea bites. The predominant reaction is edema (ed) in the upper part of dermis and an irregular dense inflammatory cell infiltrate (chiefly eosinophils) which is concentrated in the middle part of the dermis. H. & E., × 100, × 450 and × 450.

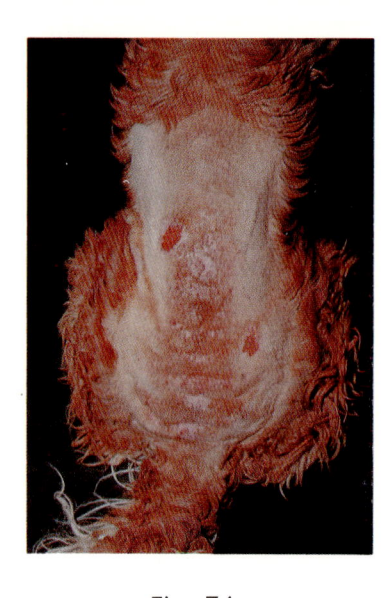

Fig. 76
Flea bites. With a long-standing infestation, continual self-inflicted trauma results in a chronic dermatitis on lower median part of back. This type of lesion is seen in the late summer and fall.

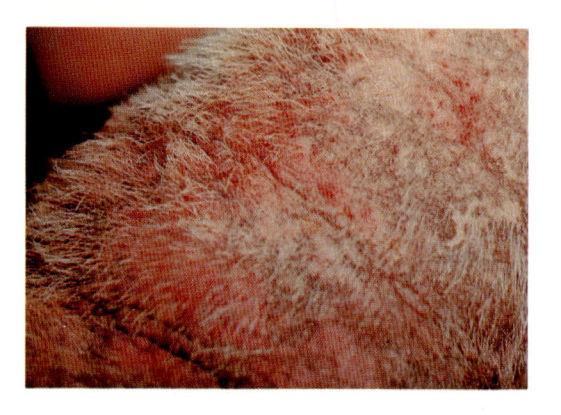

Fig. 77
Closer view of dermatitis (Fig. 76). Note hyperpigmentation, thickening and folds of skin, alopecia and erythema.

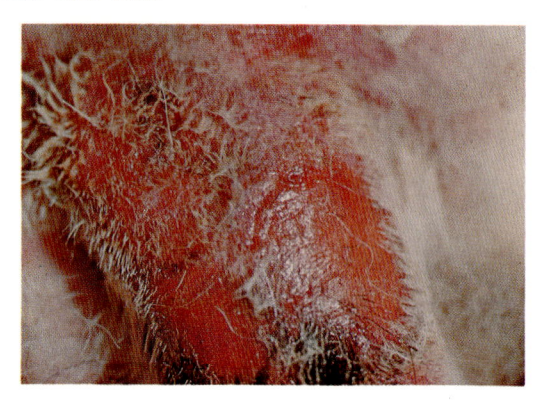

Fig. 78
Flea bite. Self-inflicted trauma results in an acute ulcerative dermatitis on tail head. This lesion usually occurs in the early part of the summer.

CHAPTER
3

PYODERMA (BACTERIAL INFECTION OF THE SKIN)

Primary pyodermas usually are caused by a single strain of bacteria (staphylococcal organisms predominantly) and occur in previously undamaged skin. Short-haired dogs, areas of friction and thin-skinned areas are particularly predisposed. (Coagulase positive, hemolytic staphylococci were isolated from lesions in Figs. 79–96.)

A. IMPETIGO

A superficial pyoderma, non-pruritic and occurring mainly on the groin.

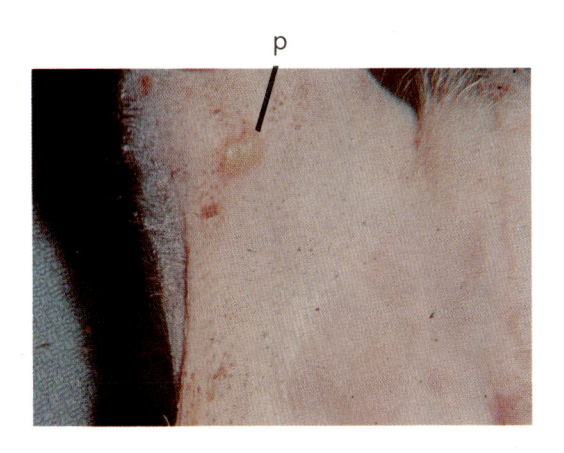

Fig. 79
A superficial pustule (p) on inner aspect of thigh. Note erythematous base.

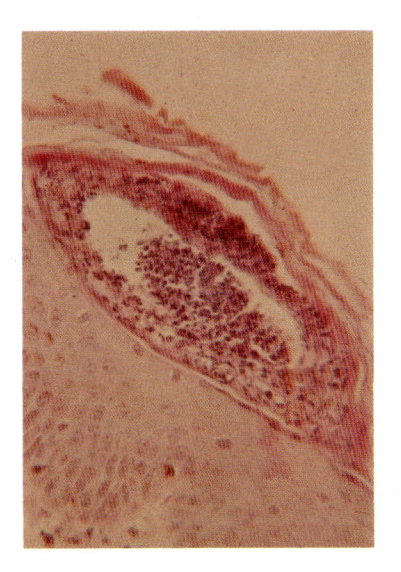

Fig. 80
Biopsy of lesion (Fig. 79). Note subcorneal abscess and acanthotic epidermis. H. & E., × 100.

B. FOLLICULITIS (SUPERFICIAL)

Infection of the hair follicle, resulting in a papular or pustular lesion which may or may not be pruritic.

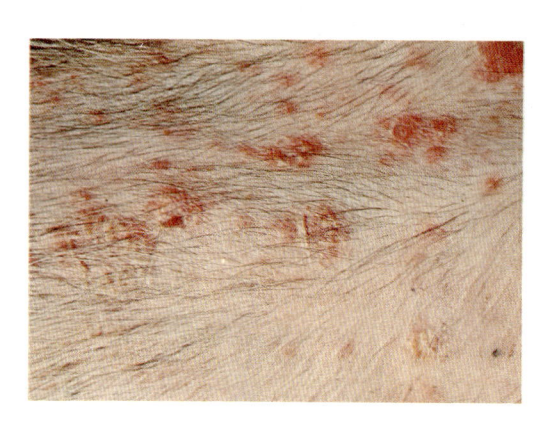

Fig. 81
Note erythematous papules, pustules and crusting (groin).

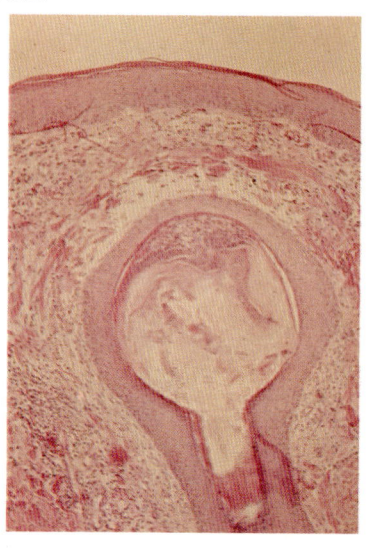

Fig. 82
Biopsy of pustule (Fig. 81). Note follicular sub-corneal abscess and perifollicular infiltrate. H. & E., × 100.

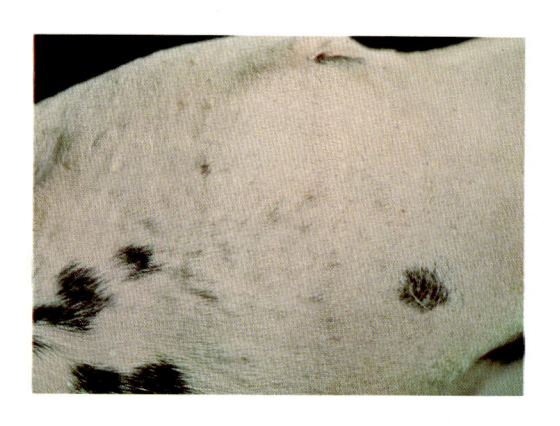

Fig. 83
Moth-eaten alopecia and palpable indurations (overlaid by disheveled hairs) on lateral aspect of face.

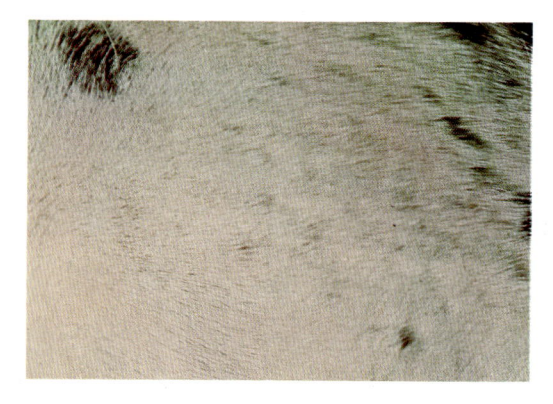

Fig. 84
Similar lesions on head.

40

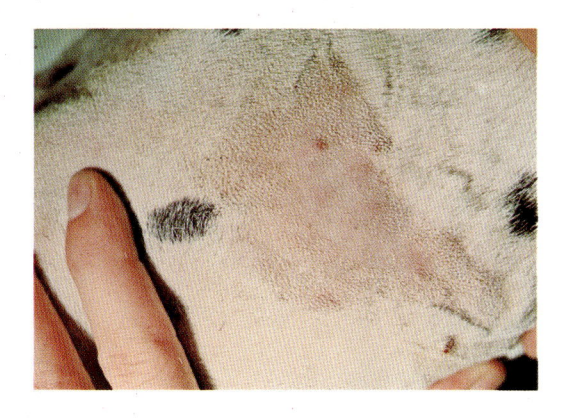

Fig. 85
A papular and pustular eruption is evident after removing hair.

C. FURUNCULOSIS

A deep infection of the hair follicle.

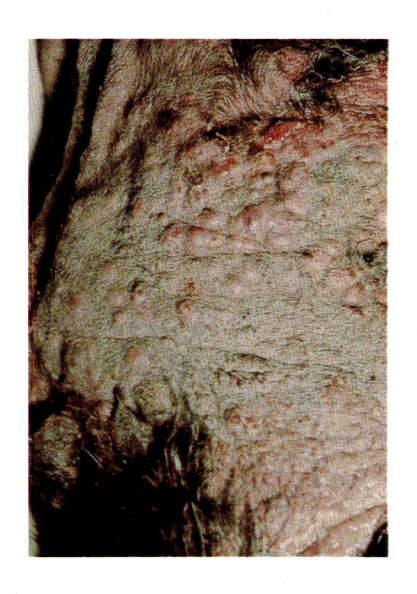

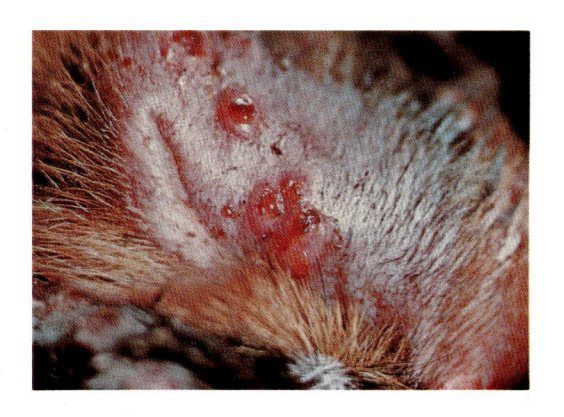

Fig. 87
Erythematous nodules on pinna. Note ulceration on summit of lesions.

Fig. 86
A cluster of erythematous nodules on groin. Pus can be expressed from these lesions.

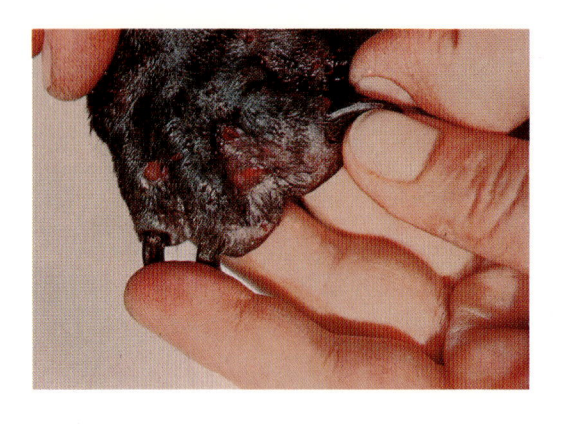

Fig. 88
Interdigital furunculosis. Most of the lesions have ulcerated.

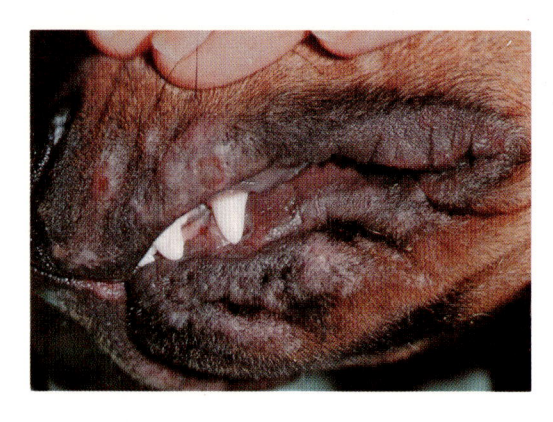

Fig. 89
Labial furunculosis.

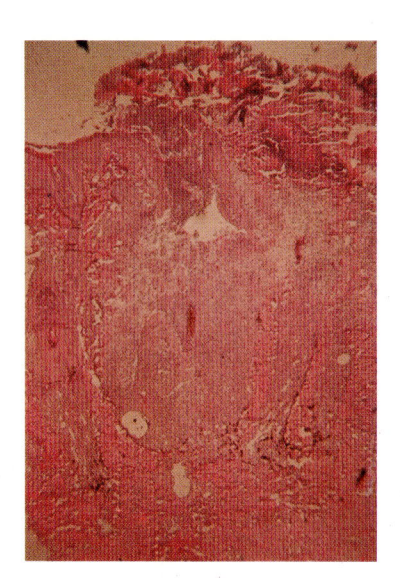

Fig. 90
Biopsy of furuncle (Fig. 86). The follicle is destroyed by a deep abscess—note inflammatory exudate discharging from follicular orifice. H. & E., × 35.

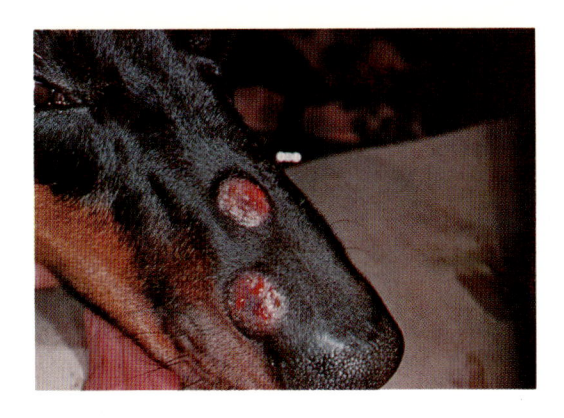

Fig. 91
Erythematous and ulcerated plaques on nose.

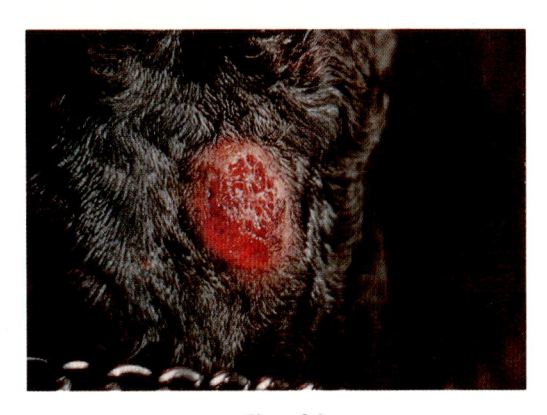

Fig. 92
Erythematous and ulcerated plaque on ventral aspect of neck.

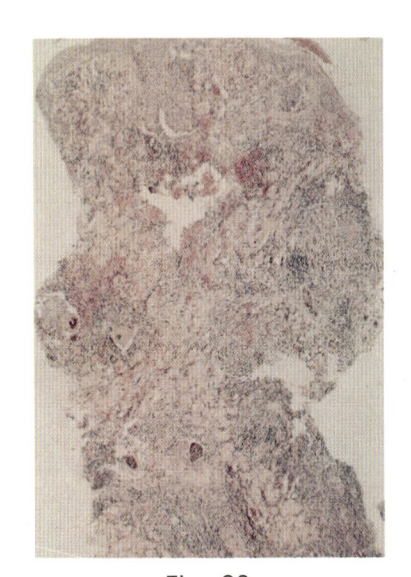

Fig. 93
Biopsy of lesion (Fig. 92). Note dense inflammatory cell infiltration and hemorrhage throughout dermis. H. & E., × 35.

D. HIDRADENITIS SUPPURATIVA

A staphylococcal pyoderma involving apocrine structures with lesions occurring on the abdomen (predominantly) and face.

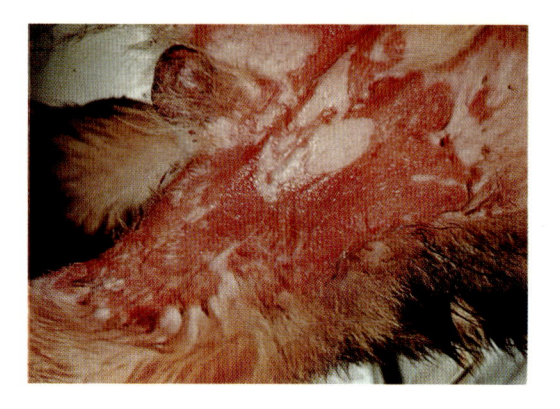

Fig. 94
Erythematous, suppurative, moist plaques on groin.

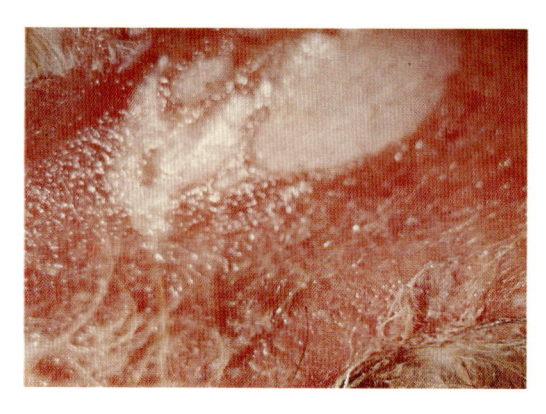

Fig. 95
A closer view of lesion (Fig. 94).

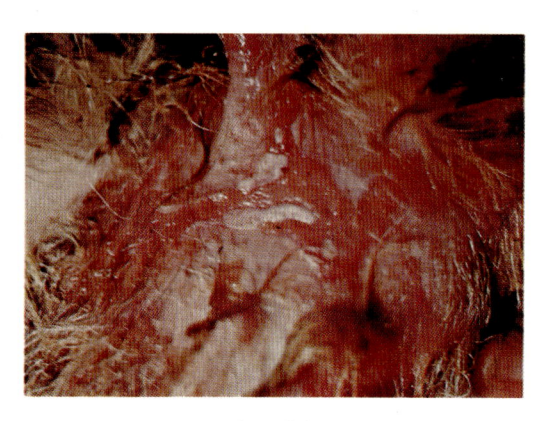

Fig. 96
Serpiginous lesion on axilla.

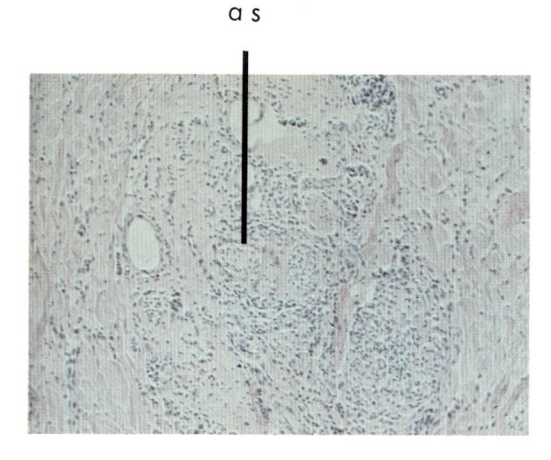

Fig. 97
Biopsy of lesion (Fig. 96). The epidermis (not shown) is ulcerated and replaced by inflammatory crust. In the lower aspect of dermis and subcutis, a subacute inflammatory infiltrate aggregates around and in apocrine structures (a s). H. & E., × 100.

E. JUVENILE PYODERMA

A cutaneous staphylococcal infection involving young dogs (4–12 weeks of age) and characterized by cellulitis of the lips, regional adenopathy, otitis externa and abscesses on the trunk.

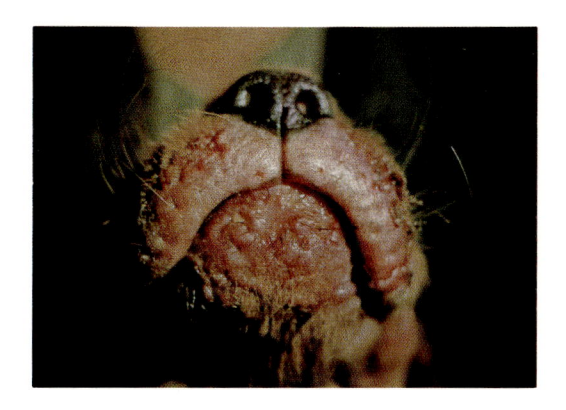

Fig. 98
The lips are swollen, hot and moist—note crusting and suppuration.

F. NECROTIZING PYODERMA
A staphylococcal infection of the skin resulting in necrosis and deep ulceration.

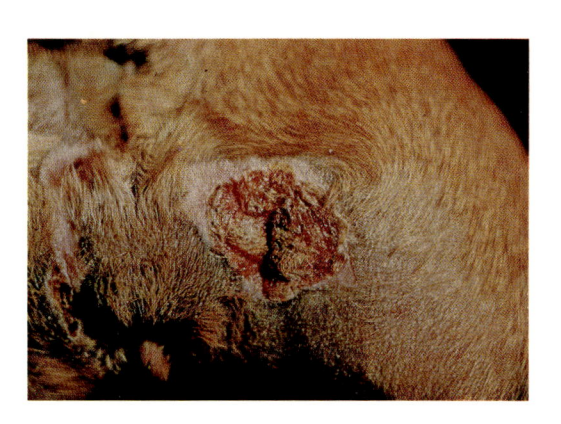

Fig. 99
A large ulcer covered by a necrotic crust.

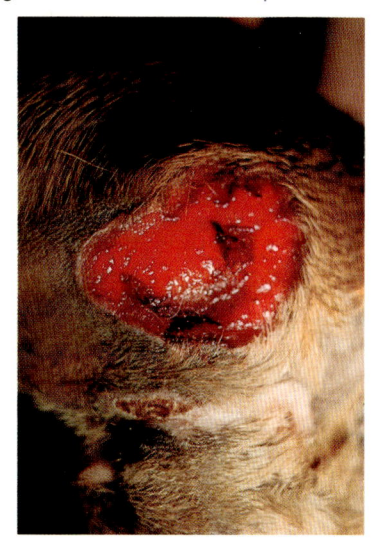

Fig. 100
Lesion (Fig. 99) after crust was removed. A deep ulcer with base of granulation tissue is evident.

G. BACTERIAL PARONYCHIA
An infection of the nail bed.

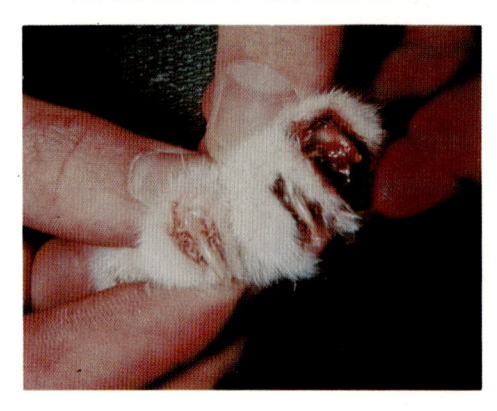

Fig. 101

(Cat.) Note suppuration and swelling of nail bed and that one nail has fallen out.

H. SECONDARY PYODERMA

Bacterial infections of the integument occurring in previously damaged skin. Often a dog or cat, in response to a pruritic sensation, will excoriate its skin and thus predispose it to infection.

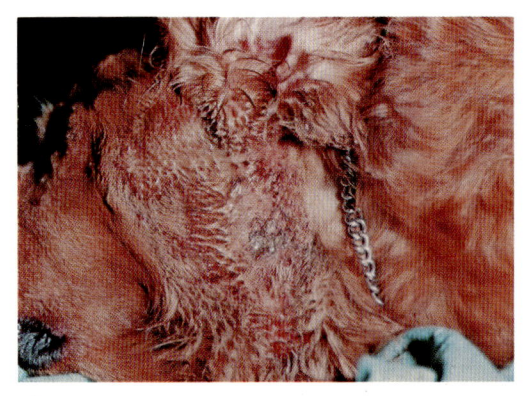

Fig. 102

A suppurative, ulcerative, infiltrated patch (hotspot, moist eczema) resulting from the dog scratching at its ear (ear mite infestation).

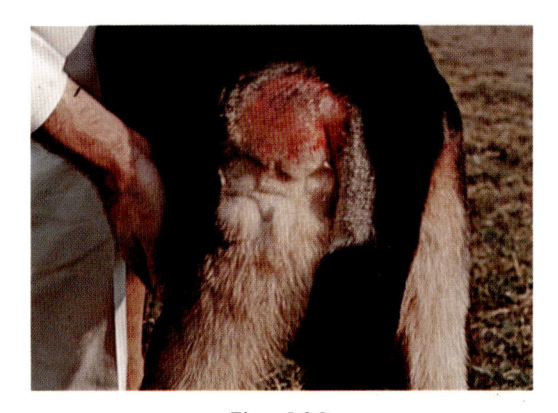

Fig. 103

An ulcerated, erythematous, alopecic, suppurative plaque resulting from the dog biting its tail head (anal gland infection).

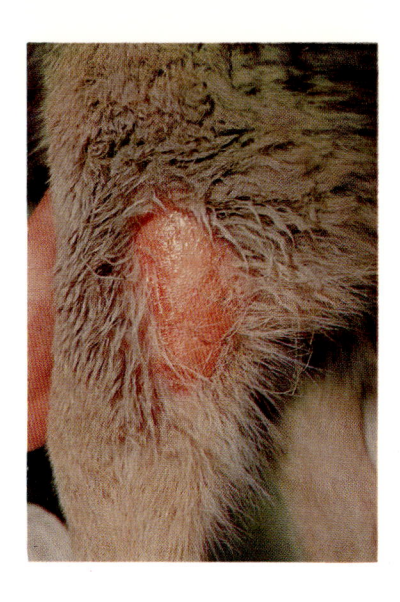

Fig. 104

A discrete, alopecic, ulcerated suppurative patch on posterior aspect of thigh resulting from self-inflicted trauma and secondary infection (animal infested with fleas).

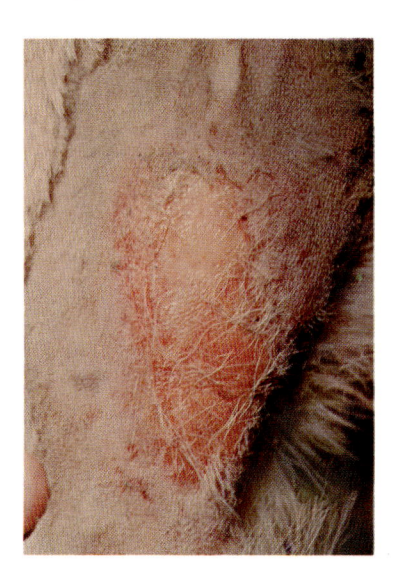

Fig. 105

Close view of lesion (Fig. 104) after removing hair.

47

Fig. 106 A

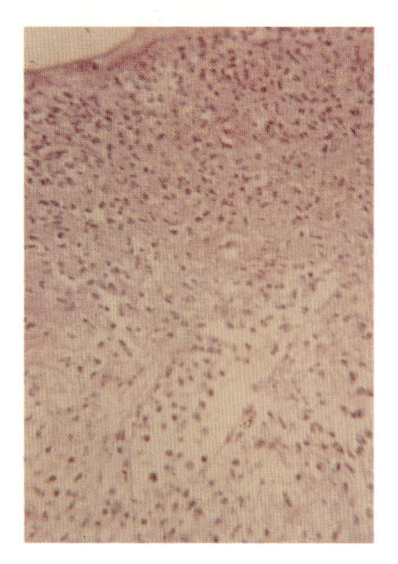

Fig. 106 B

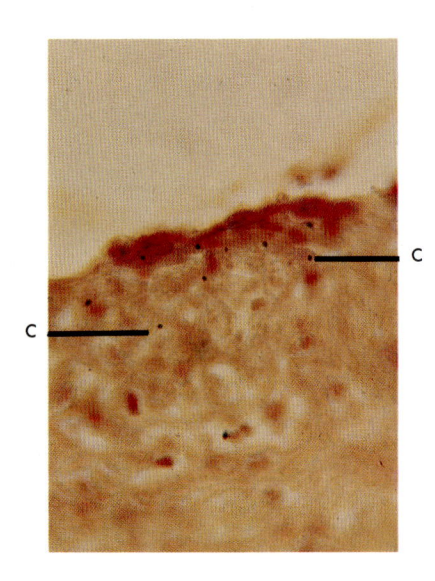

Fig. 106 C

Biopsy of lesion (Fig. 104). Note ulceration of epidermis, acute inflammatory changes in upper one-third of dermis and gram positive cocci (c) in inflammatory crust. H. & E. and Gram stain, × 100, 450 and 900.

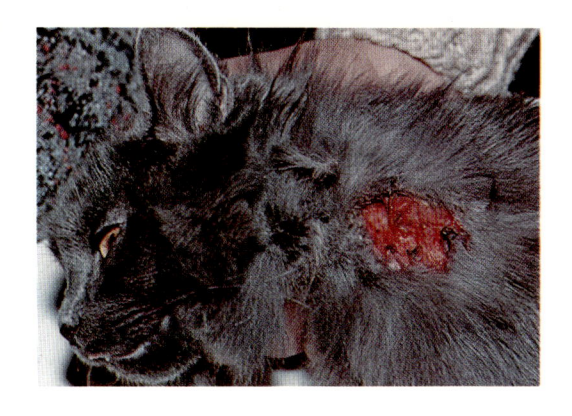

Fig. 107
(Cat.) A sorely inflamed ulcerative lesion resulting from scratching (cat infested with fleas).

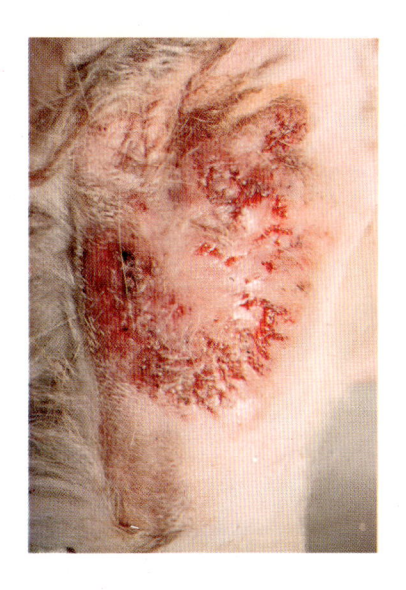

Fig. 108
A secondarily infected callus (elbow)—Note multiple draining tracts.

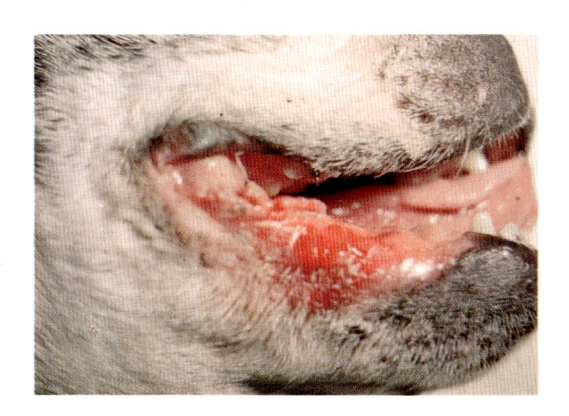

Fig. 109
A secondarily infected lip fold. Note ulcerative and erythema.

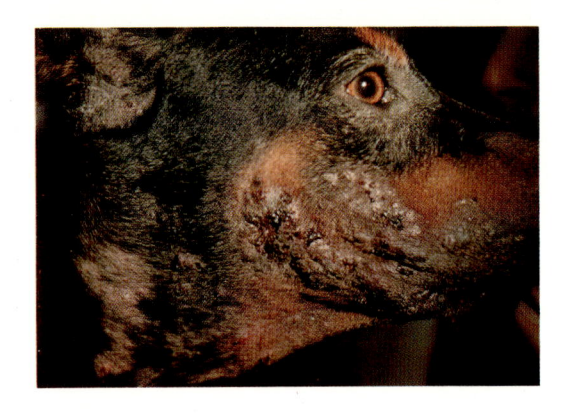

Fig. 110
Furunculosis associated with demodectic mange.

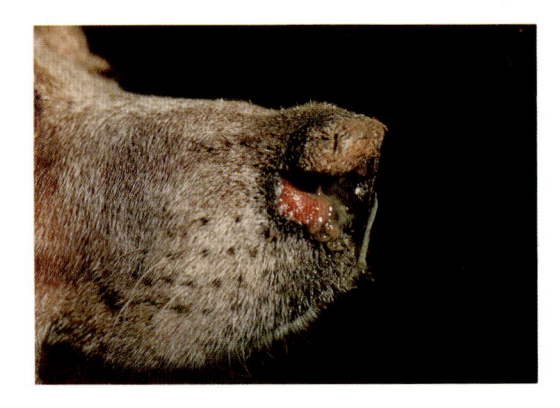

Fig. 111
Infectious eczematoid dermatitis. Ulceration of the nares resulting from a chronic purulent nasal discharge.

CHAPTER
4

SPECIFIC INFECTIONS WITH CUTANEOUS MANIFESTATIONS

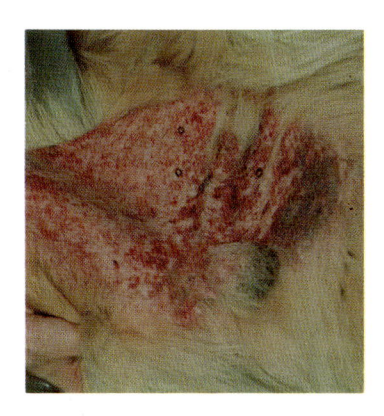

Fig. 112
Leptospirosis. Purpuric macular eruptions on groin occurring during the course of leptospirosis.

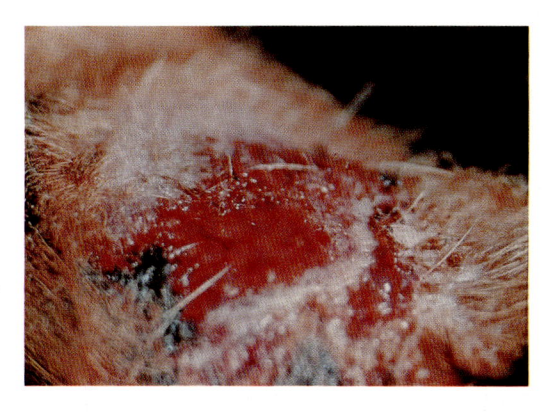

Fig. 113
Hard pad disease. Hardening of the pads associated with distemper-like viral infection.

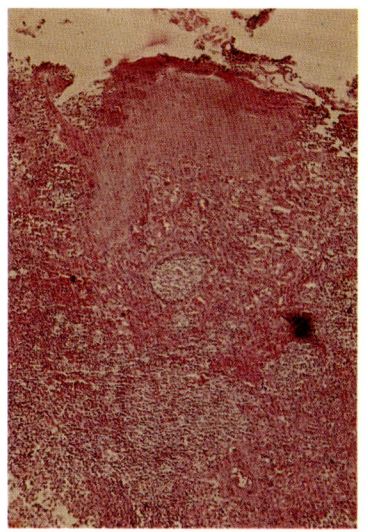

Fig. 114
North American blastomycosis. Ulcer on lateral tarsus.

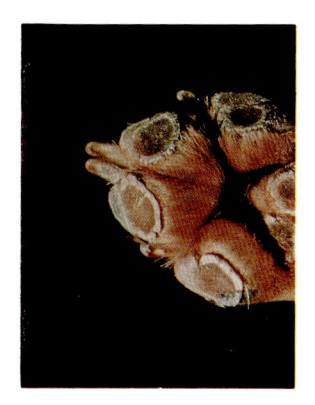

Fig. 115
North American blastomycosis—Biopsy of lesion (Fig. 114). Note alternate acanthotic and ulcerated epidermis; and dense inflammatory infiltrate in dermis. H. & E., × 68.

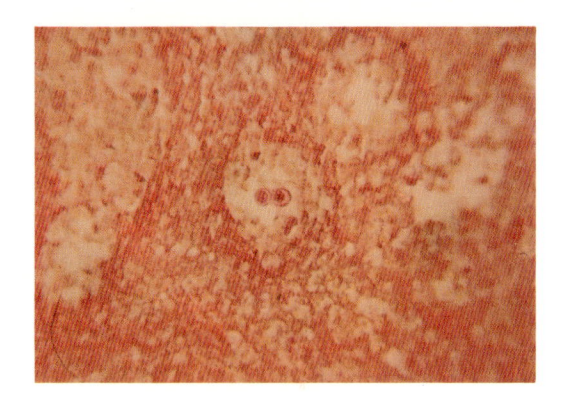

Fig. 116
North American blastomycosis—Biopsy of lesion (Fig. 114). Note double contoured budding bodies in dermal abscess. PAS × 650.

Fig. 117
Nocardiosis. A punched-out ulcer on the chest.

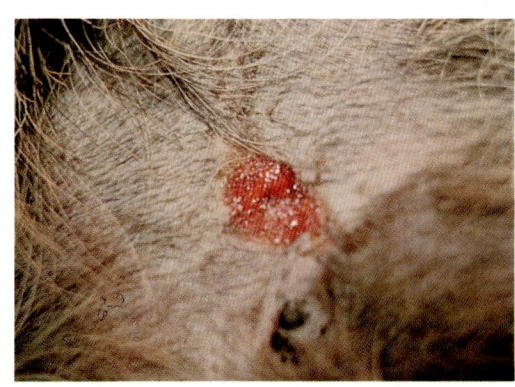

Fig. 118 A

Fig. 118 B

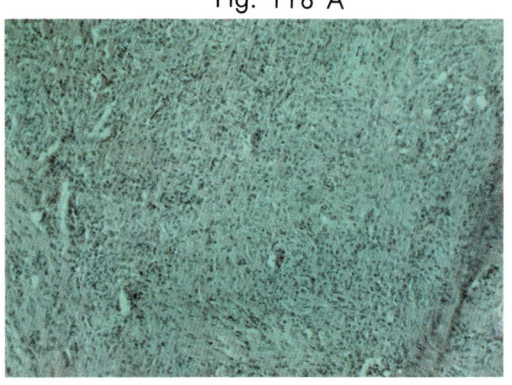

Fig. 118 C

Nocardiosis. Biopsy of lesion (Fig. 117). Tangled indistinct colonies (c) of branching filaments in necrotic cellular debris (n c d) and surrounded by a mixed chronic inflammatory reaction (C). H. & E., × 100, 1000 and 100.

CHAPTER
5

SCABIES

A pruritic, transmissible dermatitis of dogs caused by *Sarcoptes scabiei*, var. canis. A polymorphic eruption occurs predominantly on the pinna, face, ventral aspect of neck, abdomen and extremities.

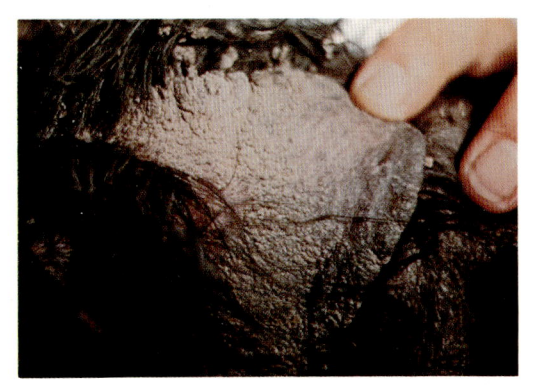

Fig. 119 A 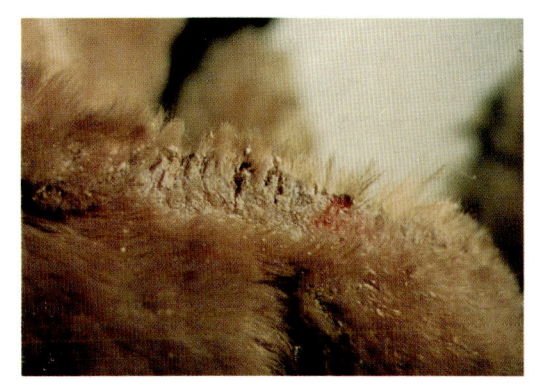   Fig. 119 B

Crusting on the pinna is a characteristic sign.

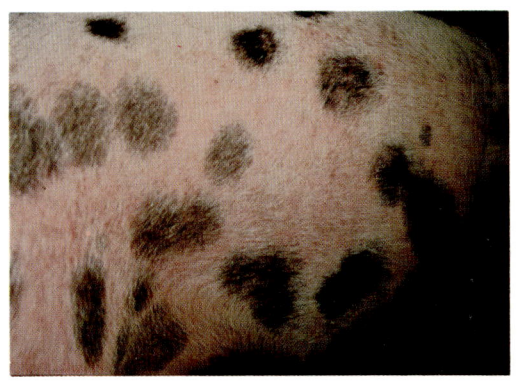

Fig. 120
An erythematous macular and papular eruption on the lateral aspect of trunk.

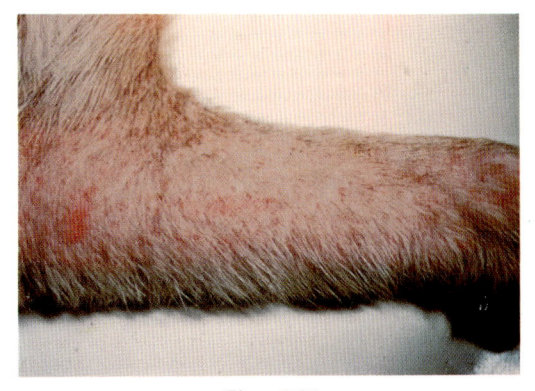

Fig. 121
Erythematous papules and pustules on inner aspect of forearm.

Fig. 122

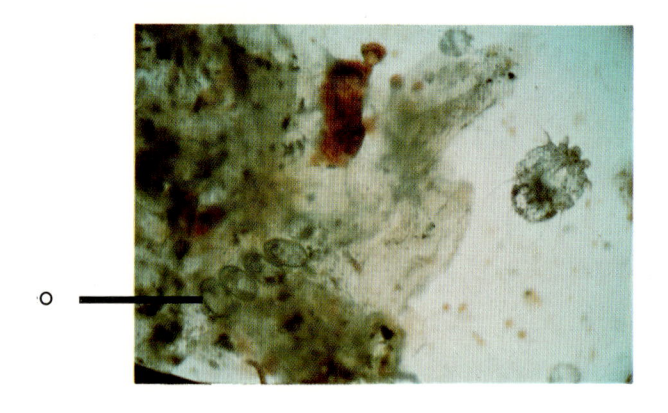

Sarcoptic mites and ova (o) as observed microscopically in skin scraping. × 100.

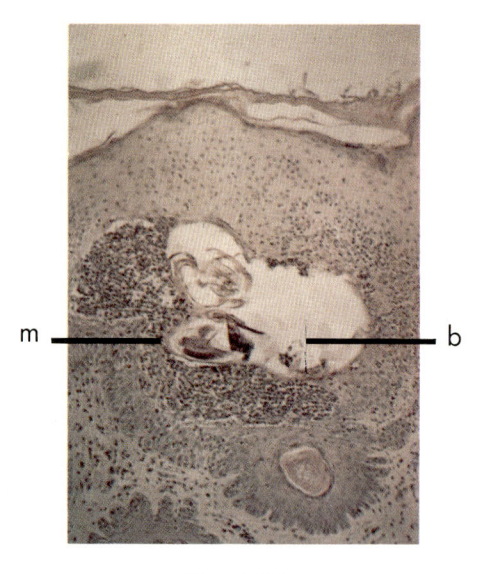

Fig. 123

Biopsy of erythematous papular lesions (Fig. 120). The epidermis is acanthotic and contains a burrow (b) within which is a mite (m) and an infiltrate of eosinophils. H. & E., × 100.

CHAPTER
6

DEMODECTIC MANGE

A non-contagious disease of young dogs (less than a year) caused by *Demodex folliculorum* var. canis. The localized form of the disease is characterized by patches of alopecia on the head, trunk and extremities with minor inflammatory changes. Pruritus usually is absent.

The generalized form of the disease is characterized by alopecia, seborrhea crusting and furunculosis. Only the ventral abdomen is spared usually. Pruritus often is present.

LOCALIZED

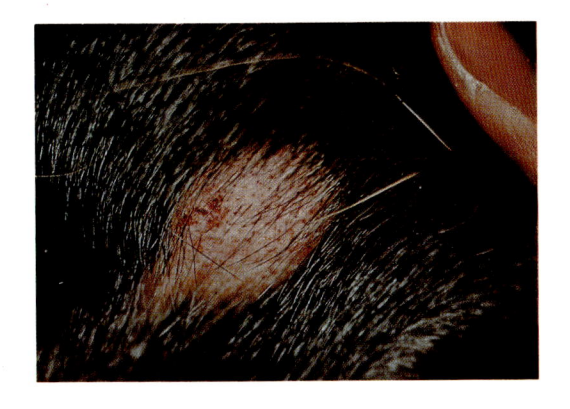

Fig. 124
A patch of alopecia on the face. Note minimal inflammatory reaction.

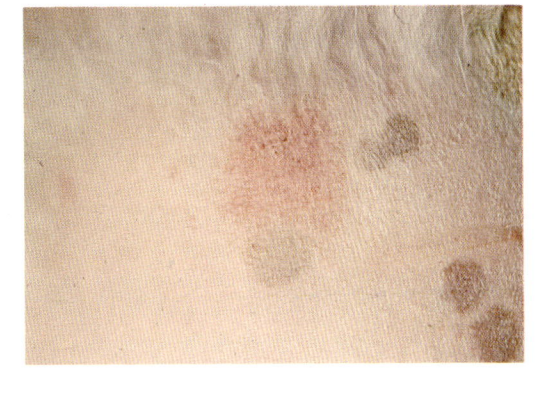

Fig. 125
An erythematous and scaling patch on chest (hair has been removed for visualization of lesion).

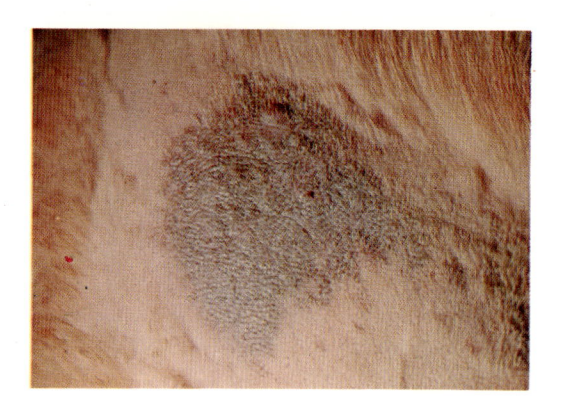

Fig. 126
A discrete hyperpigmented alopecic patch. Note follicular plugging.

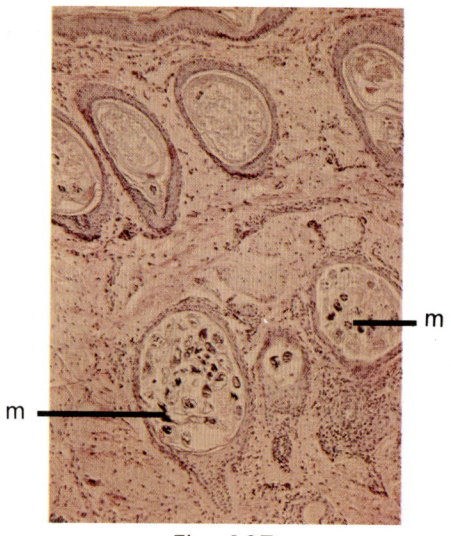

Fig. 127
Biopsy of lesion (Fig. 124). The epidermis is acanthotic and there is a minimum of inflammatory infiltration in the dermis. The follicles are filled with an excess of keratotic material and large numbers of demodectic mites (m). H. & E., × 100.

GENERALIZED

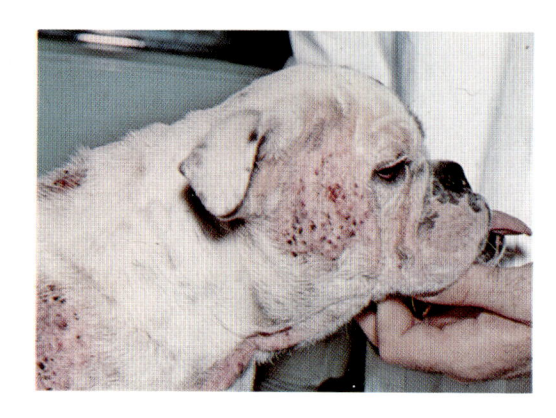

Fig. 128
Multiple erythematous furuncular plaques on face and trunk. Most of the furuncles have ulcerated.

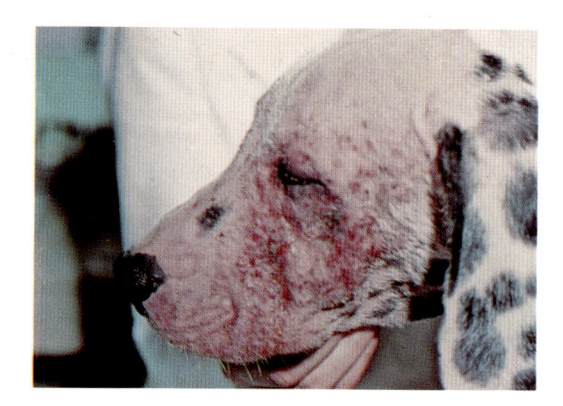

Fig. 129
Furuncular lesions on a moist erythematous base.

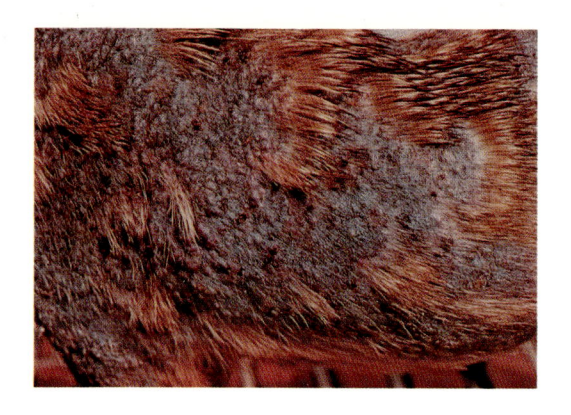

Fig. 130
Alopecia, hyperpigmentation and furunculosis on lateral aspect of the chest.

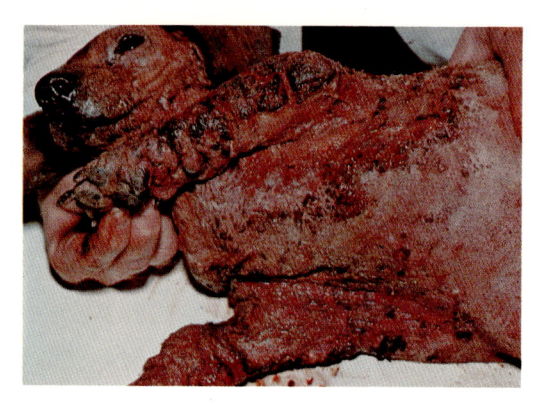

Fig. 131
Ulceration, suppuration and crusting on axillae and extremities.

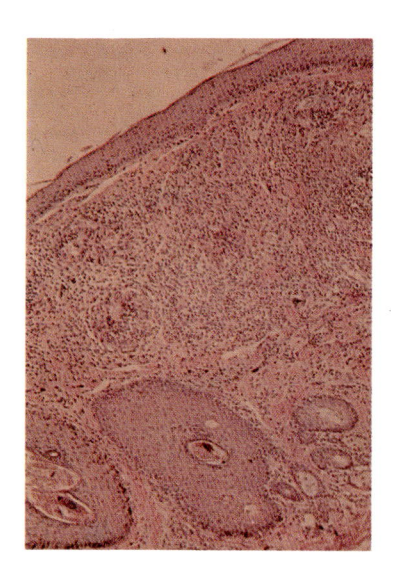

Fig. 132
Biopsy of lesion (Fig. 130). The epidermis is acanthotic and in the upper aspect of the dermis, there is follicular destruction and a polymorphonuclear and histiocytic cell infiltrate. H. & E., × 100.

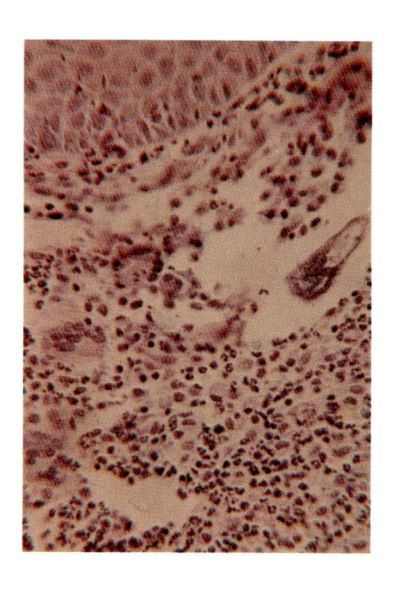

Fig. 133
Biopsy of lesion (Fig. 130). A demodectic mite is free in dermis. Note infiltration of polymorphonuclear leukocytes, histiocytes and giant cells. H. & E., × 450.

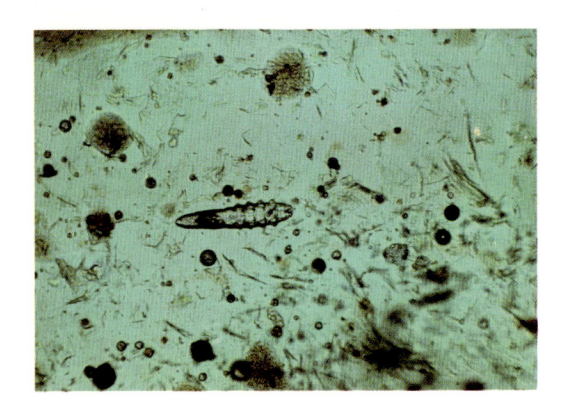

Fig. 134
Demodectic mite as seen in skin scraping. × 100.

CHAPTER
7

RHABDITIC DERMATITIS

A nematode (*R. strongyloides*) dermatosis of dogs with a polymorphic eruption involving the extremities, and ventral and lateral aspects of the trunk.

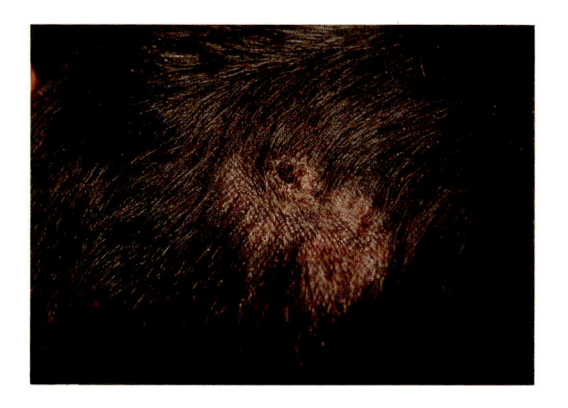

Fig. 135
A patch of alopecia on the lateral aspect of the trunk showing hyperpigmentation, erythema and crusting.

Fig. 136
Biopsy of lesion (Fig. 135). The epidermis is acanthotic and the follicles in the upper one-half of the dermis contain numerous nematodes (n) and keratotic material. An inflammatory infiltration aggregates around the appendages in the deeper aspects of the dermis. H. & E., × 35.

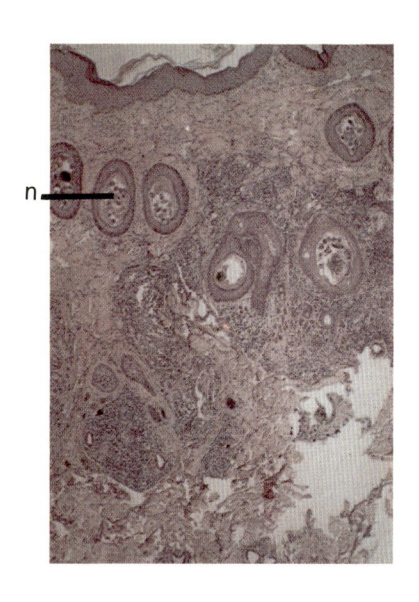

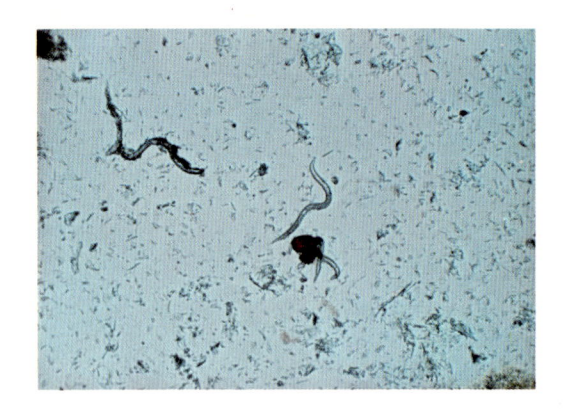

Fig. 137
Skin scraping of lesion (Fig. 135). *R. strongyloides* × 35.

CHAPTER
8

CHEYLETIELLA PARASITIVORAX DERMATITIS

An acaridal (C. parasitivorax) infestation of dog, cat, rabbits, squirrels, poultry, fox and man, characterized primarily by scaling and crusting. Pruritus and alopecia may or may not be present.

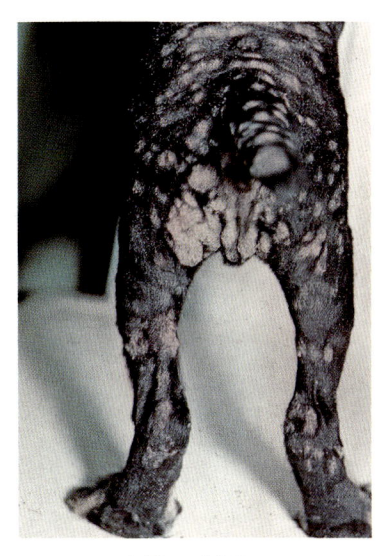

Fig. 138

Multiple discrete crusty patches on extremities and trunk.

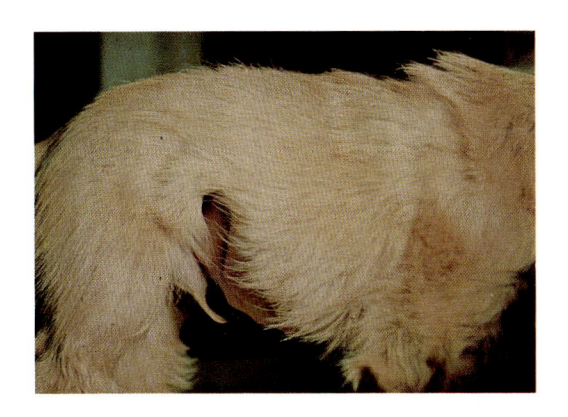

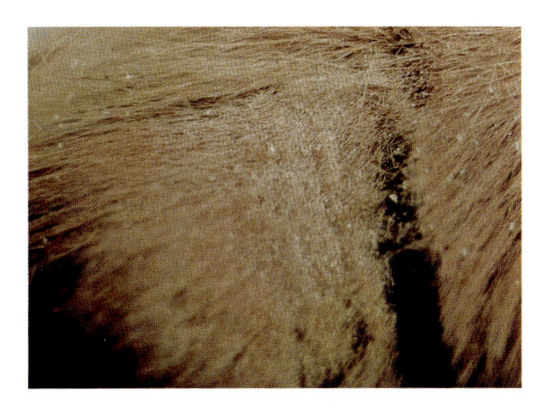

Fig. 139 A   Fig. 139 B

Before removing a patch of the hair coat, the animal manifested minimal dandruff. When the skin surface was exposed, an intense scaling process was revealed (the mite— Fig. 141—was identified in the surface scale).

61

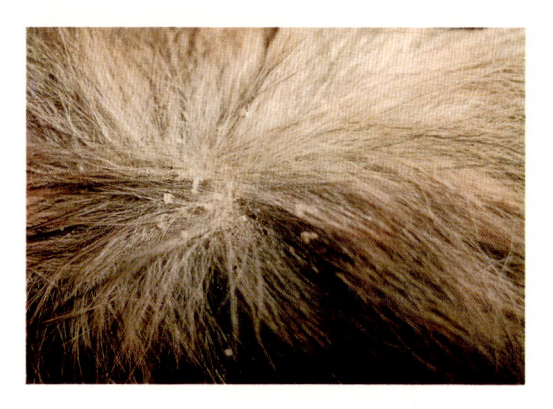

Fig. 140

Another case in which moderate scaling is the only manifestation of the infestation.

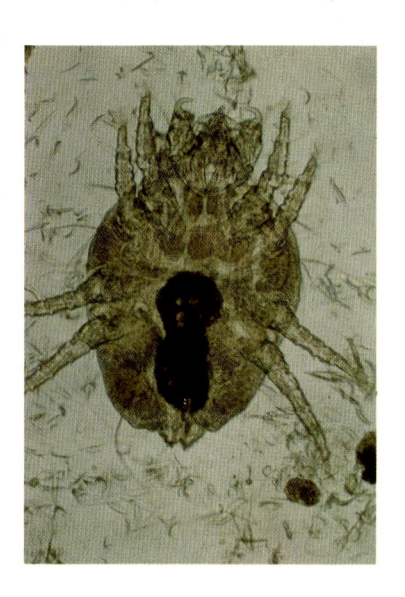

Fig. 141

Skin scraping from lesion (Fig. 124)—*Cheyletiella parasitivorax* × 100.

CHAPTER
9

NOTOEDRIC MANGE

An acarodermatitis (*N. cati*) of cats affecting primarily the ears, head, neck and lower parts of the extremities and characterized by crusting and intense pruritus.

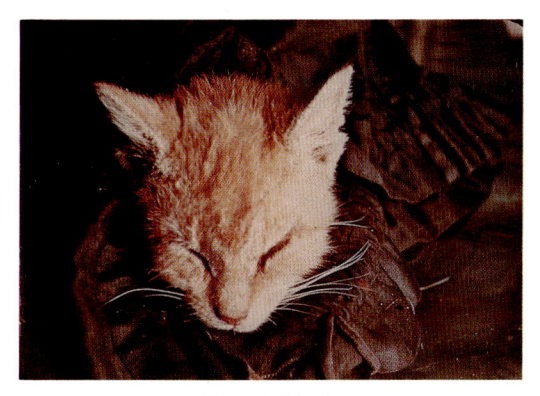

Fig. 142 A 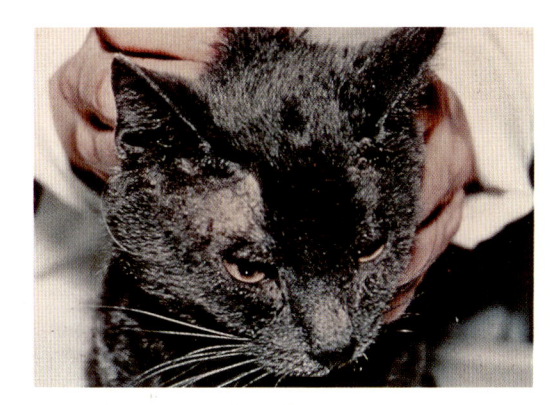   Fig. 142 B

Note alopecia and crusting on margin of ears.

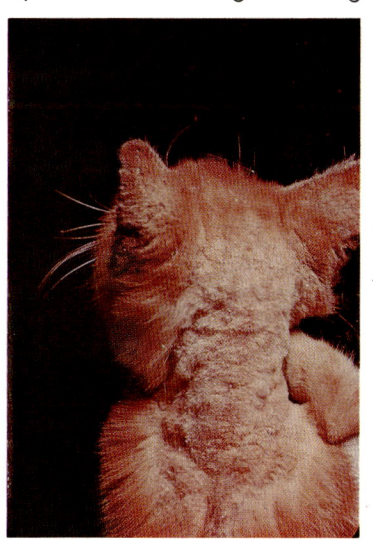

Fig. 143

Crusting on pinnae and chronic dermatitis on dorsal part of neck (hair has been removed for visualization of lesion).

CHAPTER
10

DERMATOMYCOSIS

A fungal infection of keratin caused by dermatophytes and usually characterized by an expanding circular lesion with an erythematous border. Varying inflammatory reactions may occur and the head and extremities frequently are involved.

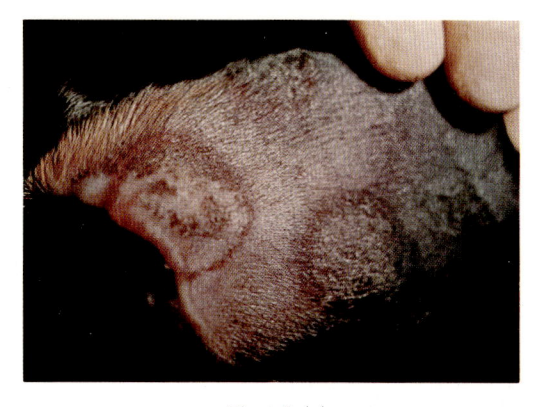

Fig. 144
Two annular lesions on pinna. Note reactive border and central scaling (*M. canis*).

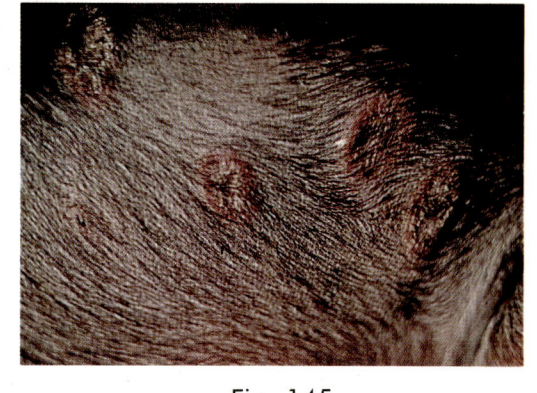

Fig. 145
Four classical lesions on abdomen (*M. canis*).

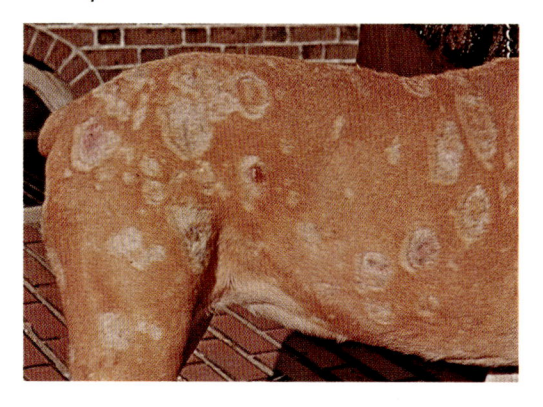

Fig. 146
Multiple circular lesions of alopecia and scaling on trunk (*M. gypseum*).

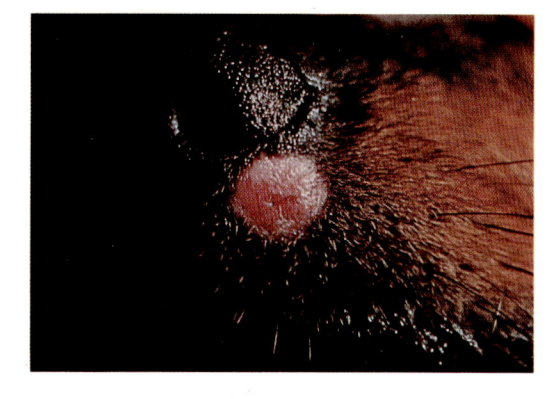

Fig. 147
A nodular lesion below muzzle (*M. canis*).

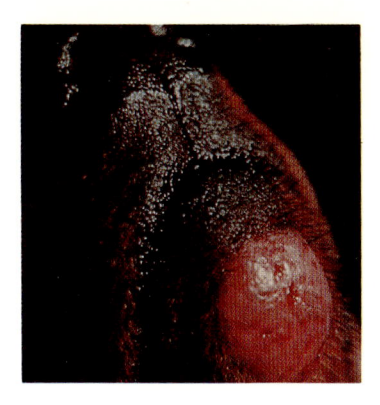

Fig. 148
A tumor-like lesion on chin *(M. canis)*—note multiple points of ulceration.

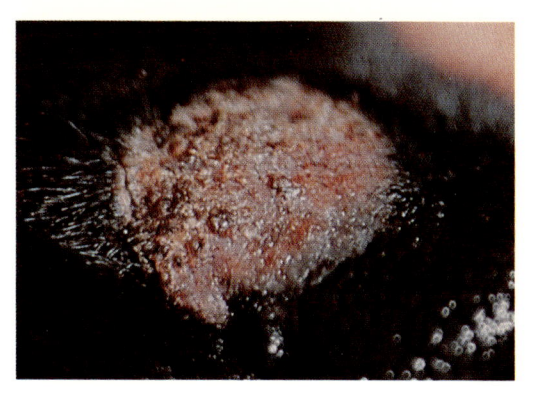

Fig. 149
A crusty alopecic lesion behind muzzle *(M. gypseum)*.

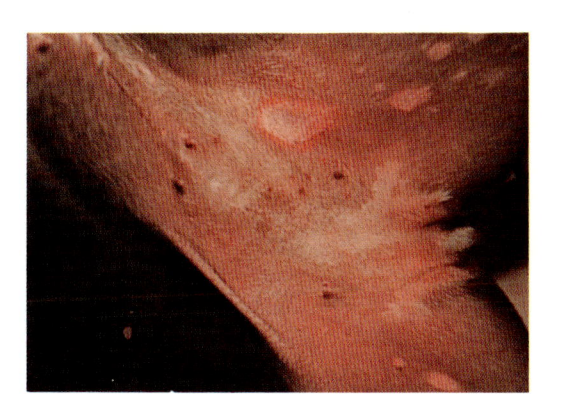

Fig. 150
Patches of alopecia with reactive borders on groin *(T. metagrophytes)*.

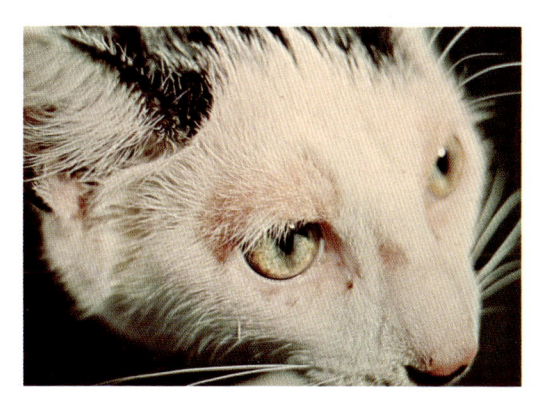

Fig. 151
(Cat). A non-discrete patch of incomplete alopecia and erythema on upper lid and a smaller lesion on lateral aspect of the nose *(M. canis)*.

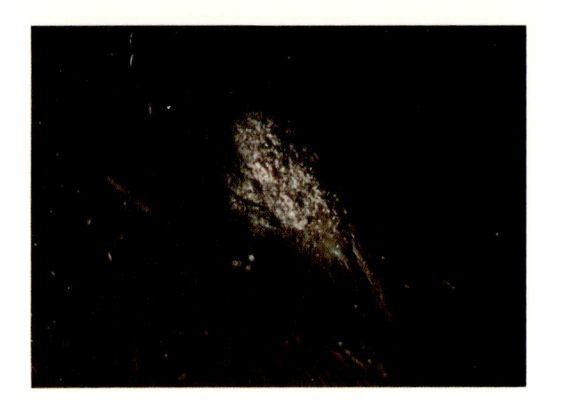

Fig. 152
(Cat). A discrete patch of alopecia, pigmentation and scaling on pinna (*M. canis*).

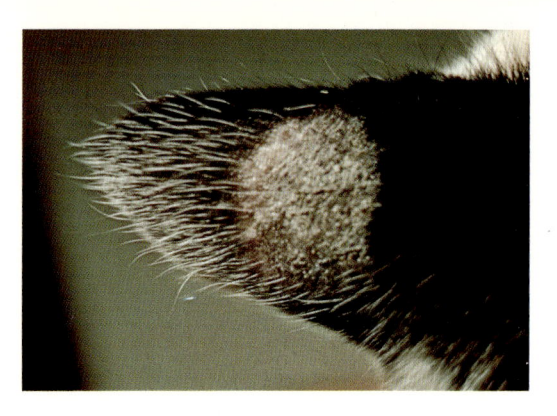

Fig. 153
(Cat). A scaling lesion on base of ear (*M. canis*).

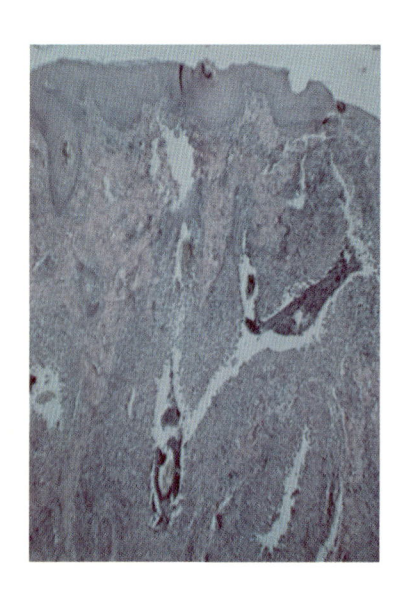

Fig. 154
Biopsy of lesion (Fig. 148). The epidermis is acanthotic and an intense acute inflammatory infiltrate aggregates around and in the follicles, eventually destroying them. H. & E., × 35.

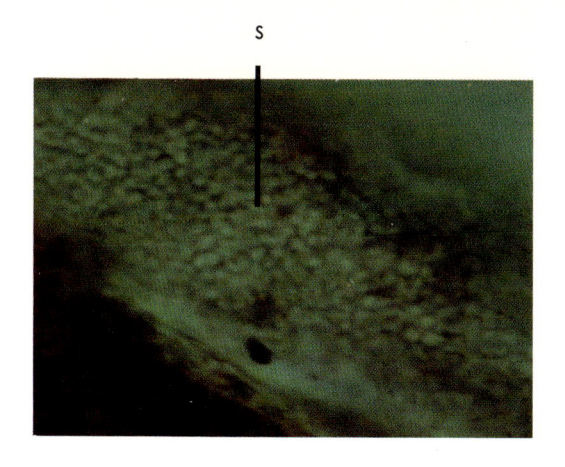

Fig. 155
Spores (s) of *M. canis* (culturally proven) on hair shaft. KOH × 400.

Fig. 156
Hyphae (h) in stratum corneum. PAS × 100.

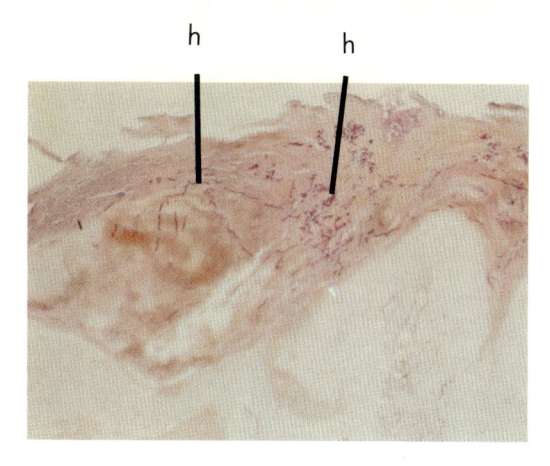

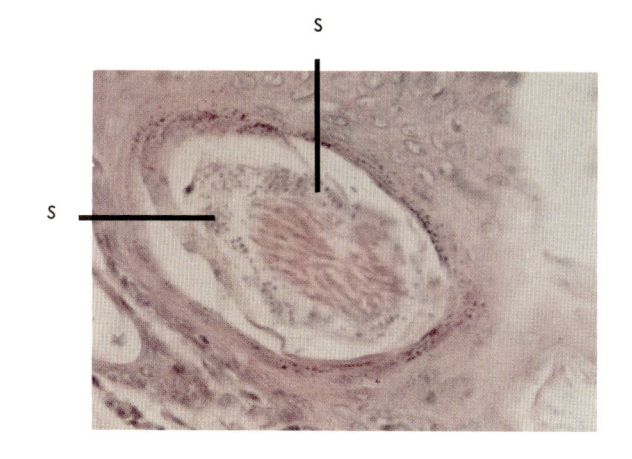

Fig. 157
Spores (s) on hair shaft within follicle. H. & E., × 100.

CHAPTER 11

MONILIASIS

An acute moist ulcerative dermatitis caused by *C. albicans*.

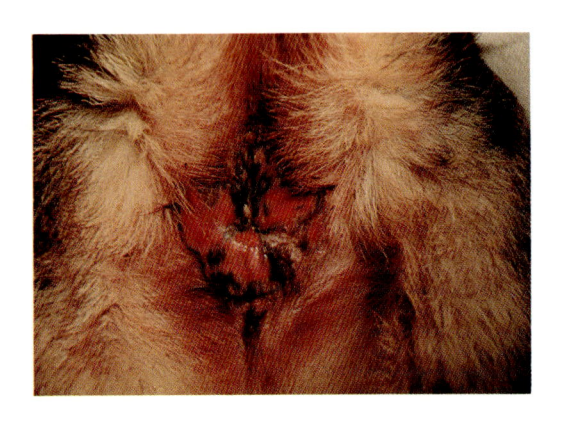

Fig. 158
A superficially ulcerated erythematous patch (perianal region).

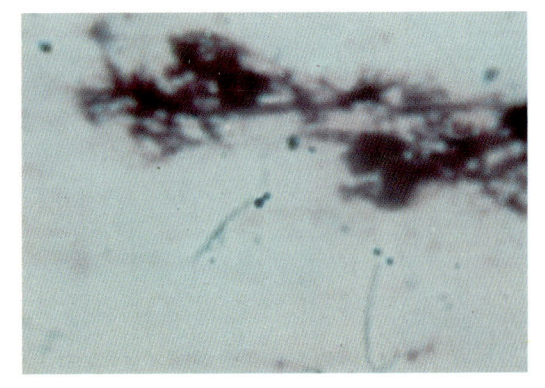

Fig. 159
Smear of lesion (Fig. 158). Note budding yeast (in center of picture). Wright's stain × 1000.

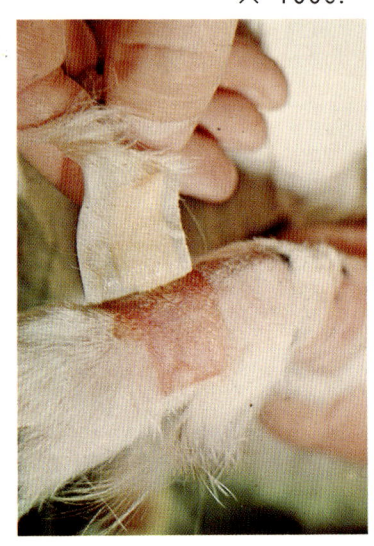

Fig. 160
Experimentally induced infection. A suppurating erythematous plaque on metacarpal area.

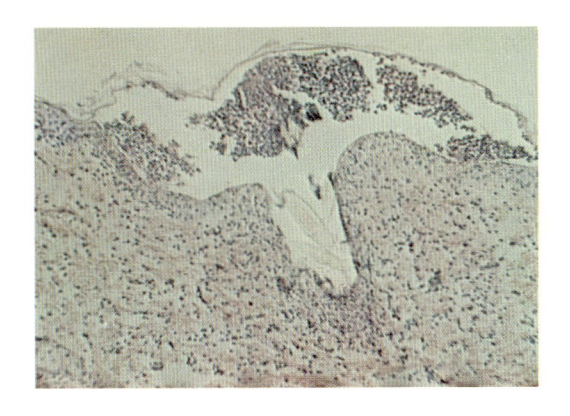

Fig. 161

Experimentally induced lesion (24 hours post-infection—Fig. 160). Note subcorneal abscess and acute inflammatory changes in upper portion of the dermis and epidermis. H. & E., × 100.

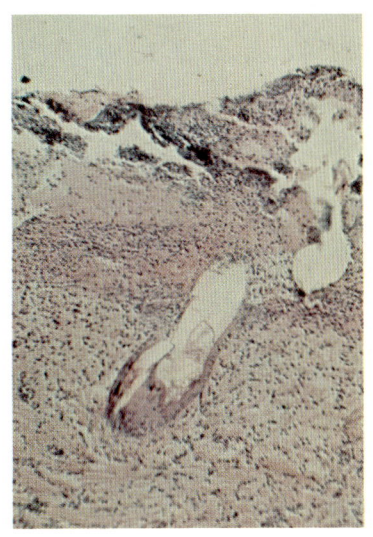

Fig. 162

Experimentally induced lesion (48 hours post-infection). Note ulceration, inflammatory crust and acute inflammatory reaction in upper part of the dermis. H. & E., × 100.

CHAPTER 12

SEBORRHEA

A disorder of the follicular sebaceous apparatus of uncertain causation characterized by scaling, crusting and alopecia. Three forms of the disease exist: a dry (sicca), oily (oleosa) and dermatitic.

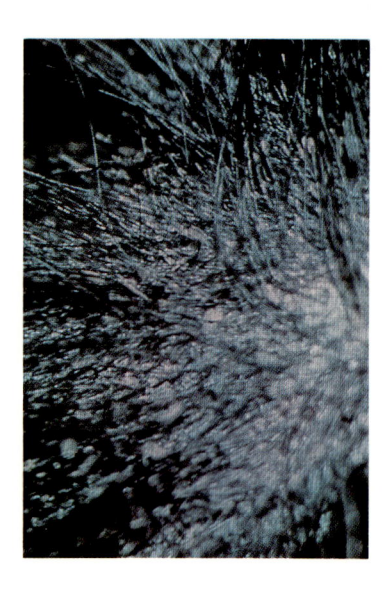

Fig. 163
Surface scaling and nit-like keratotic deposits are present on the hair shafts (pinna).

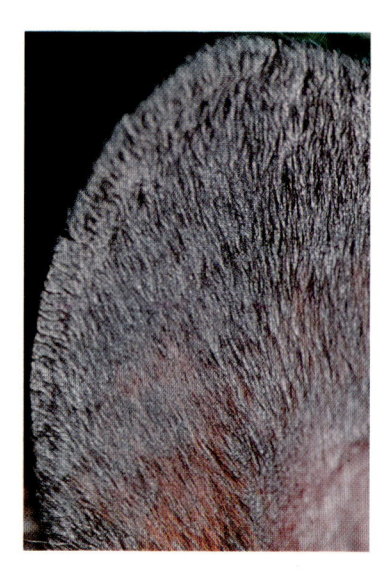

Fig. 164
The hairs on the ear margins are matted with a keratotic material.

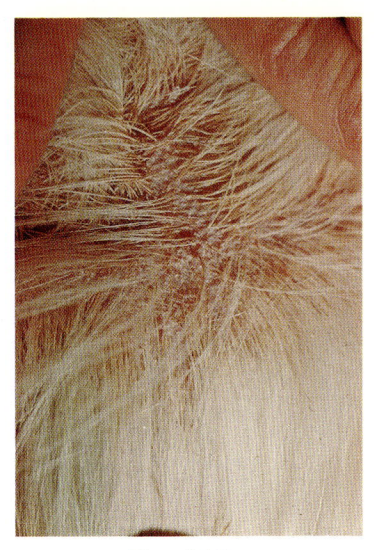

Fig. 165
Seborrhea oleosa. The hairs are stained yellow by an excess of sebaceous material.

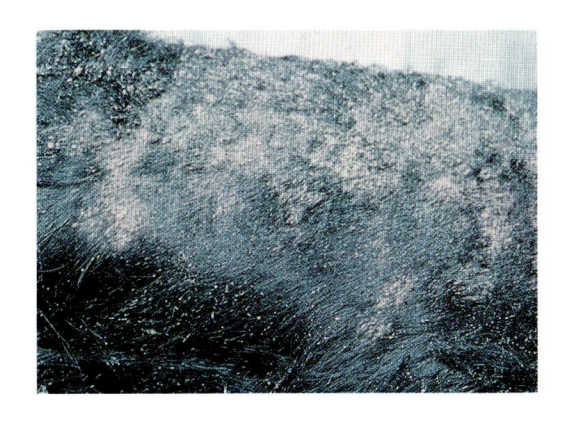

Fig. 166
Scaling and crusting on back (hairs have been removed for visualization of lesion).

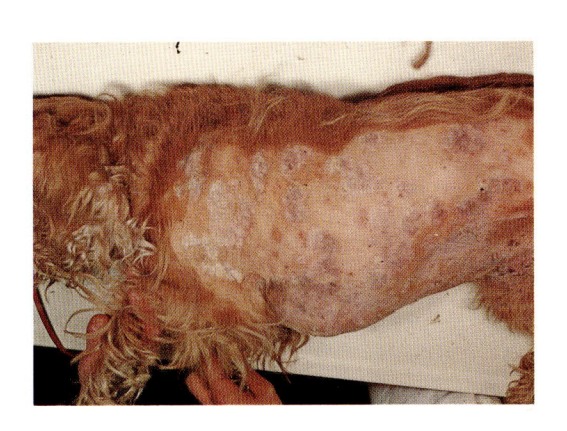

Fig. 167
Multiple circular hyperpigmented and crusty lesions on trunk (resembling ringworm). This form of seborrhea is common in blond Cocker Spaniels, Springer Spaniels and Dachshunds.

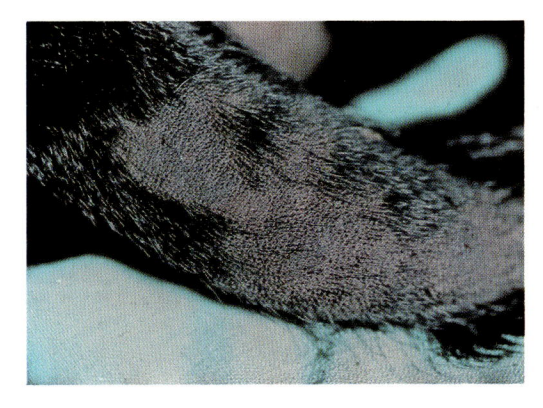

Fig. 168
Alopecia on dorsum of tail (near tail head) often occurs in association with other seborrheic skin changes.

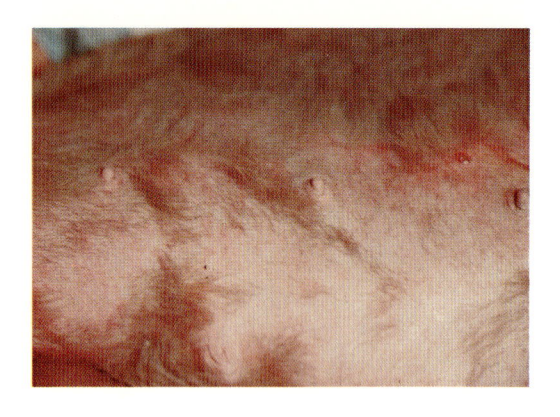

Fig. 169
A linear erythematous plaque on hair line and an erythematous macular and papular eruption on abdomen.

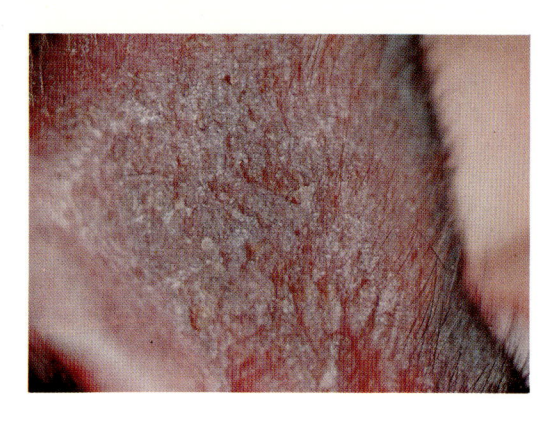

Fig. 170
Seborrheic dermatitis. Scaling and crusting on a dermatitic base (pinna).

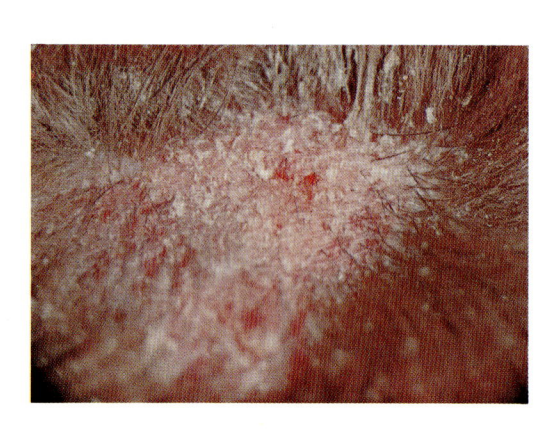

Fig. 171
Seborrheic dermatitis. Note alopecia, erythema, scaling and oily encrustation of peripheral hair (median back).

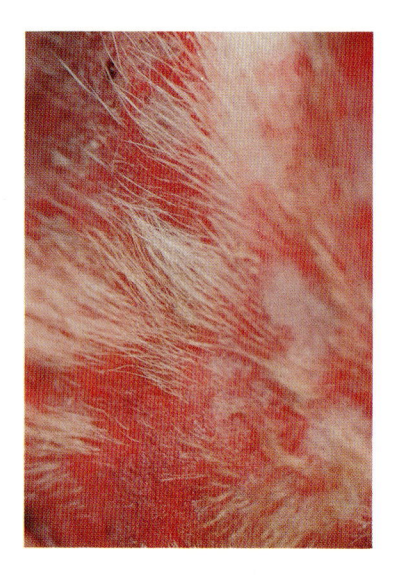

Fig. 172
Seborrheic dermatitis. Erythematous patches on abdomen.

CHAPTER 13

FACIAL KERATOSIS

A dermatosis of uncertain origin (usually occurring in nervous dogs) and characterized by symmetrical alopecia, scaling or crusting lesions around the eyes, nose or other parts of the face.

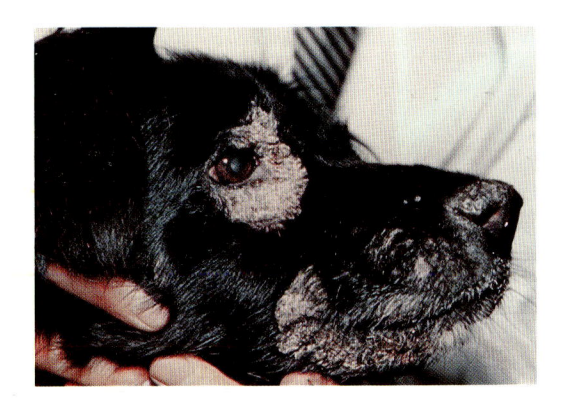

Fig. 173
Note discrete alopecic and crusty patches around the eyes and lips.

FOLLICULAR KERATOSIS

A rare hereditary dermatosis characterized by firm papules covered with horny crusts, seated in the follicular orifices and symmetrically distributed on the trunk, neck and head.

Fig. 174
Note gray follicular papules on lower part of the back.

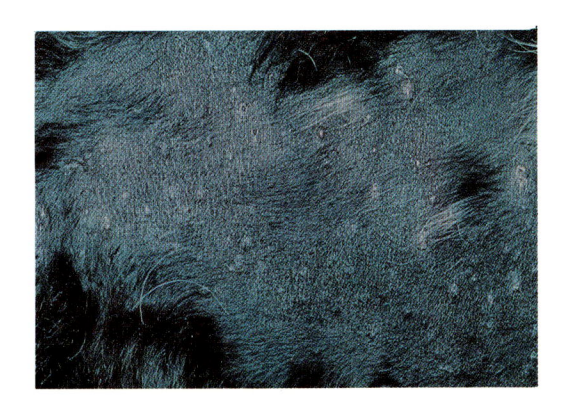

CHAPTER
14

THALLIUM INTOXICATION

A poisoning with a rodenticide characterized by severe systemic manifestations and variety of cutaneous lesions—alopecia (principally), crusting and erythema.

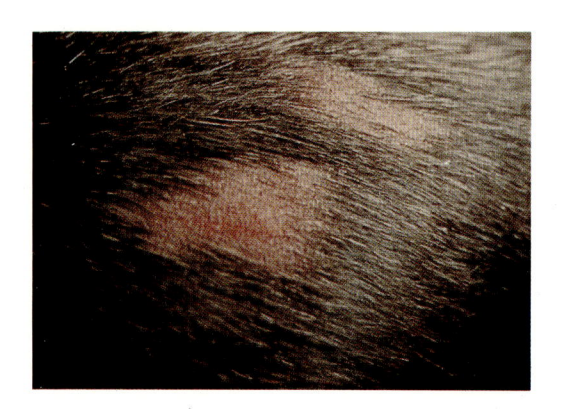

Fig. 175
Patches of alopecia produced by epilating telogen hairs. Alopecia is the result of the toxic effect of the poison on the hair bulb. The entire pelage is affected in contrast to the hormonal alopecias which primarily involve the hair of the trunk.

Fig. 176
Note generalized alopecia and absence of dermatitis. Hairs present can be epilated with ease.

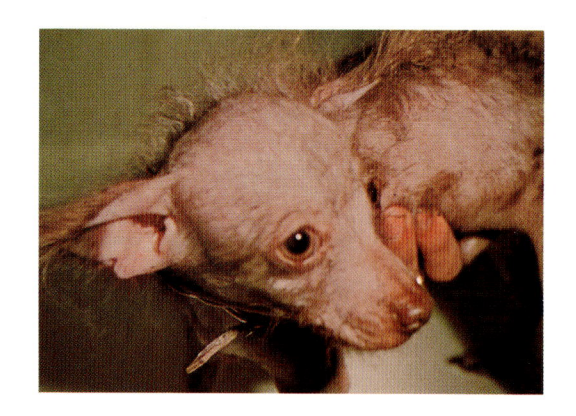

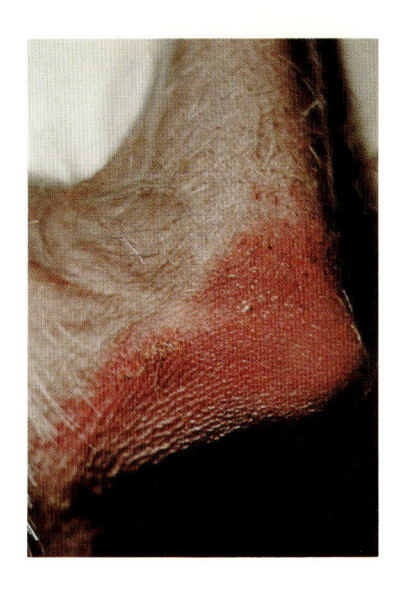

Fig. 177
An erythematous patch on inner aspect of elbow. Similar reactions may be seen on other intertriginous sites.

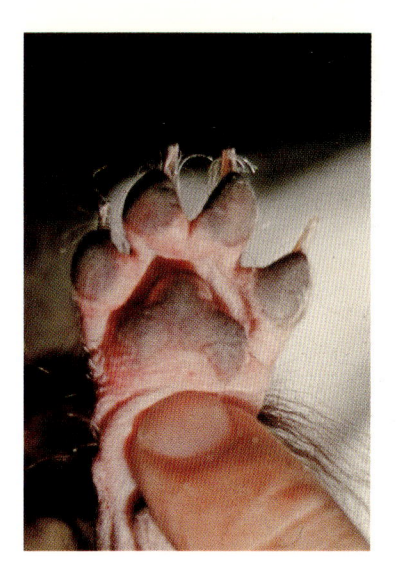

Fig. 178
Interdigital erythema.

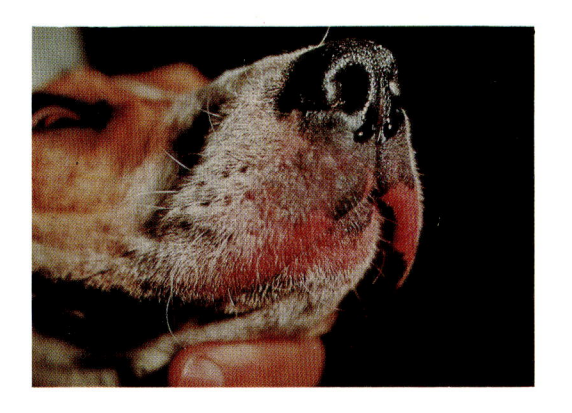

Fig. 179
Erythema on lips.

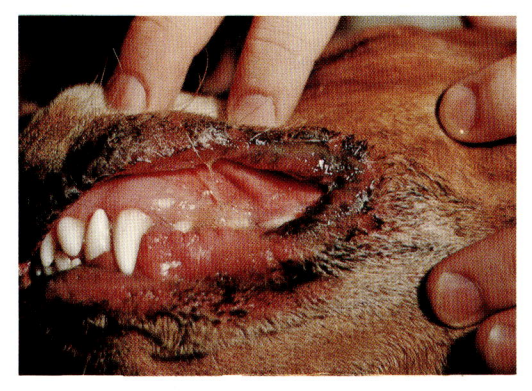

Fig. 180
Ulceration and crusting on lips.

75

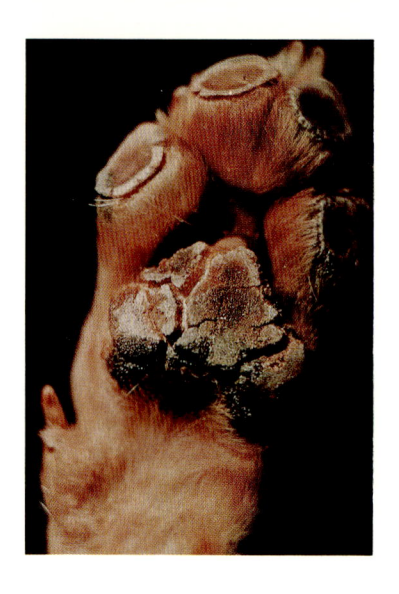

Fig. 181
The pads often become hard and fissured.

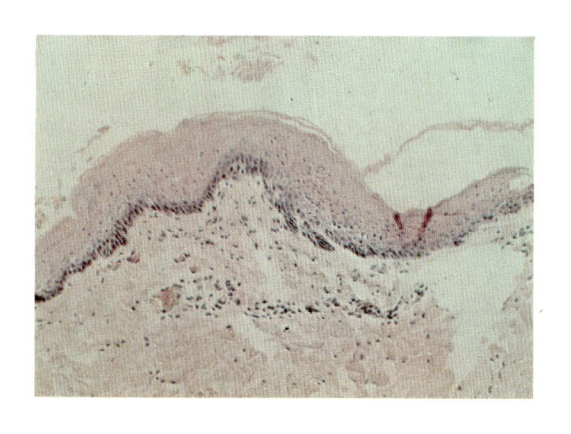

Fig. 182
Biopsy of lesion (Fig. 177). Note parakeratotic layer. H. & E., ×100.

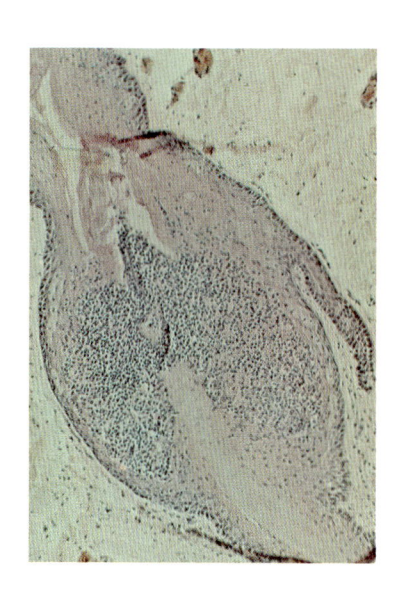

Fig. 183
Biopsy of lesion (Fig. 179). Note parakeratosis and spongiform pustule in telogen follicle. H. & E., ×100.

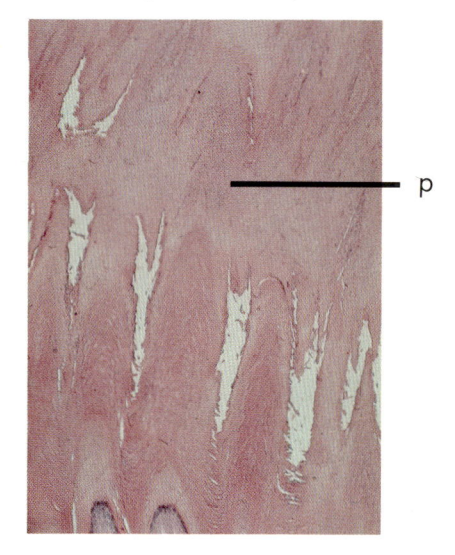

Fig. 184
Biopsy of lesion (Fig. 181). Note massive hyperkeratotic and parakeratotic (p) layer. H. & E., × 35.

CHAPTER
15

CALLUS

Intermittent pressure and/or friction on skin areas over bony prominences result in hyperplastic horny "growths" which are of no clinical importance unless they become infected.

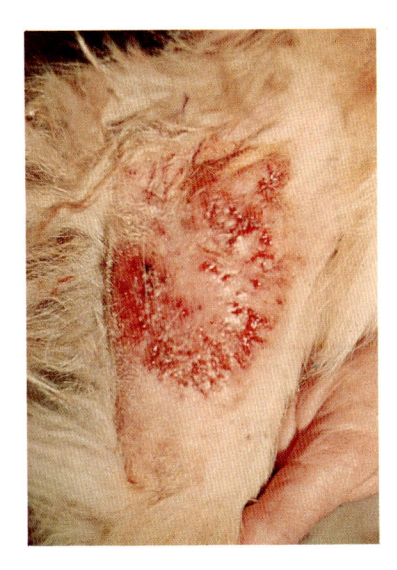

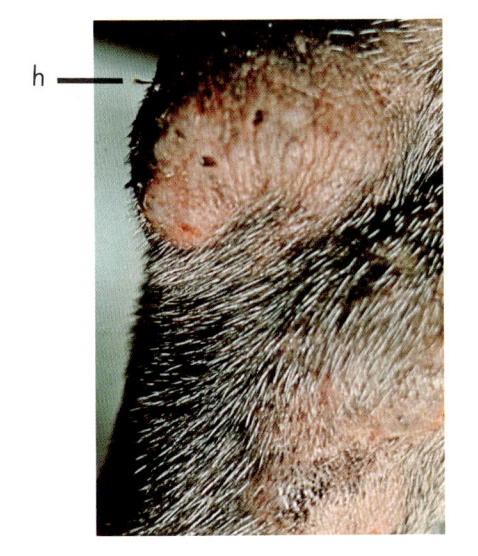

Fig. 185
An infected callus on lateral aspect of the elbow with multiple draining tracts (after clipping).

Fig. 186
Cellulitis on point of hock. Impacted hairs (h) have been expressed.

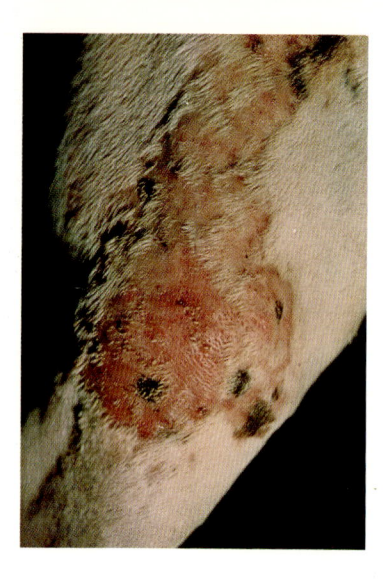

Fig. 187
An erythematous plaque on lateral aspect of leg.

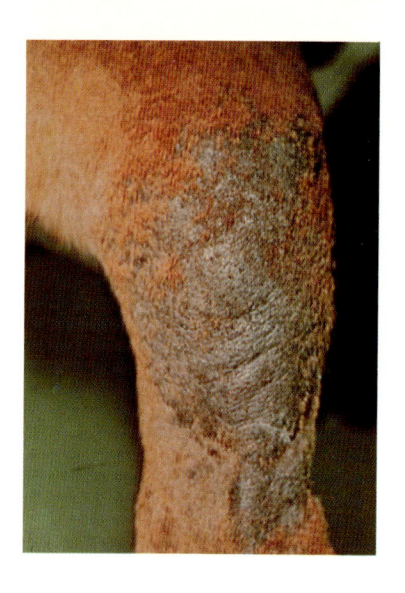

Fig. 188
Hyperpigmented plaque on lateral part of leg. Impacted hairs and pus can be expressed manually.

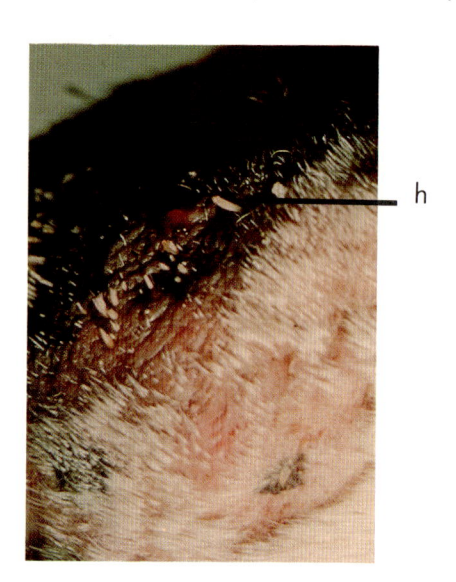

Fig. 189
Impacted hairs (h) have been expressed from lesion (Fig. 187).

CHAPTER 16

ACRAL-PRURITIC NODULE

A pruritic tumor-like lesion on the carpus (usually) or tarsus and below occurring usually in the larger short-haired breeds. Boredom or foreign bodies may be primary causative factors. The nodules often are secondarily infected.

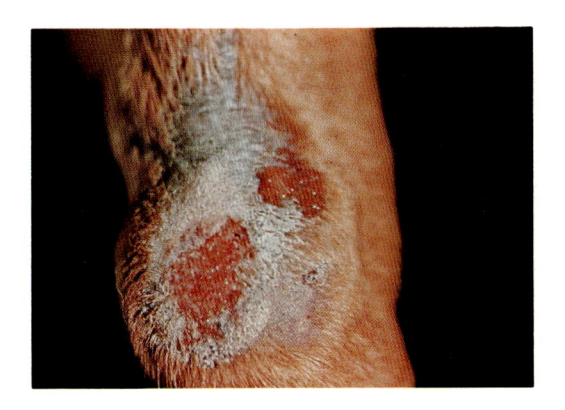

Fig. 190

A firm ulcerated nodule on anterior aspect of the carpus.

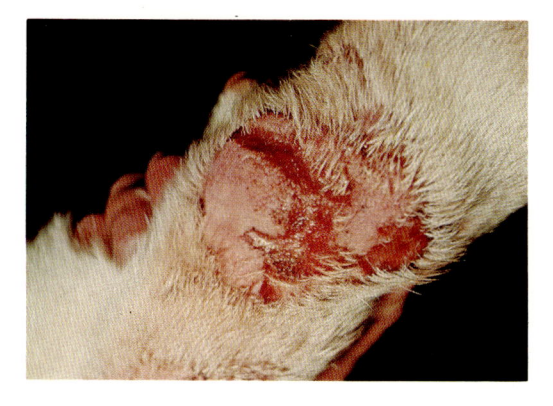

Fig. 191

A tumorous mass with ulceration on carpal area.

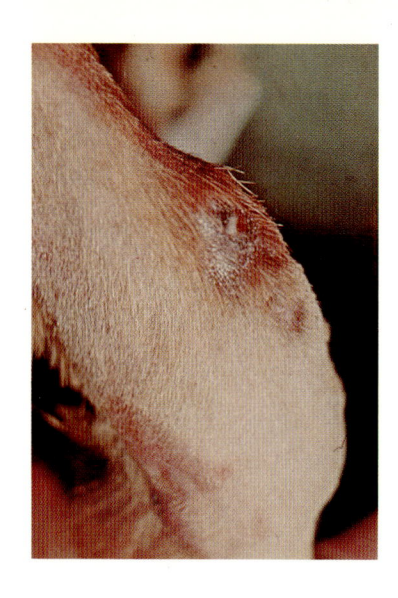

Fig. 192
An early lesion on the knee.

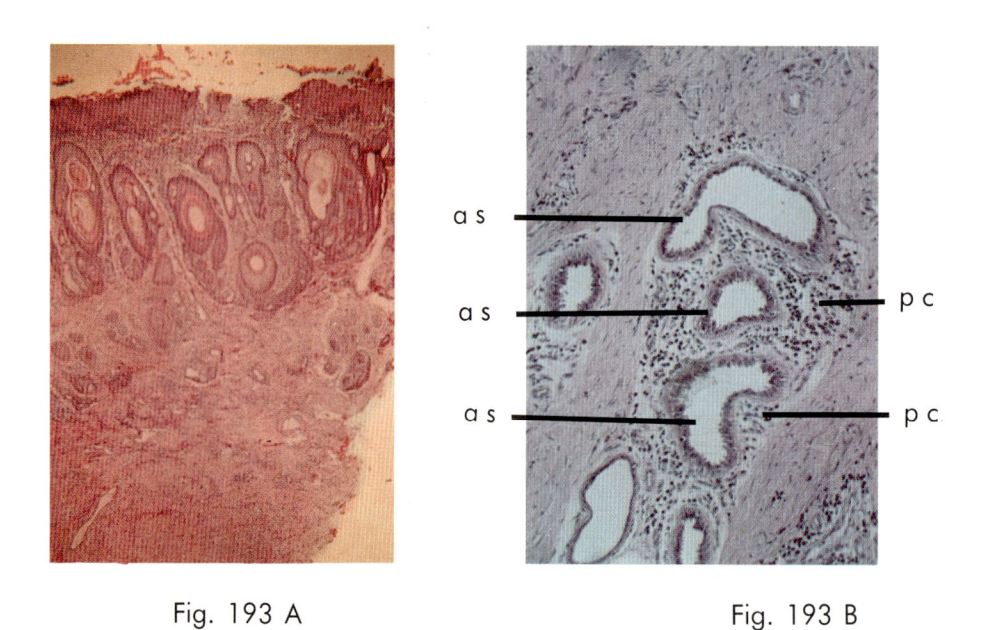

Fig. 193 A   Fig. 193 B

Biopsy of lesion (Fig. 192). The most characteristic histopathologic finding is a plasma cell (p c) infiltrate around apocrine structures (a s). Chronic inflammatory changes in the dermis and loss of the epidermis are associated. H. & E., × 35 and 100.

CHAPTER 17

SLOUGH

Necrosis of tissue from normal tissue.

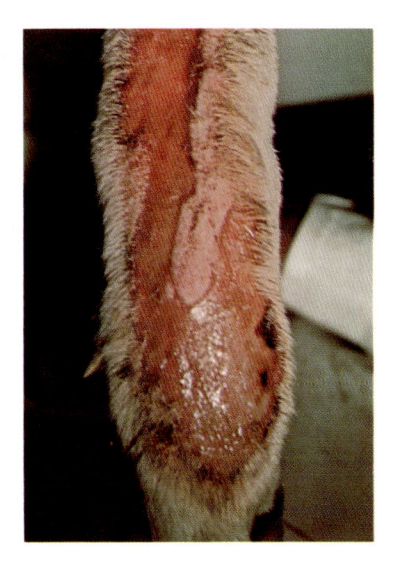

Fig. 194

An extensive deep ulcer on the anterior forearm resulting from improper intravenous injection of phthalofyne (Whipcide).

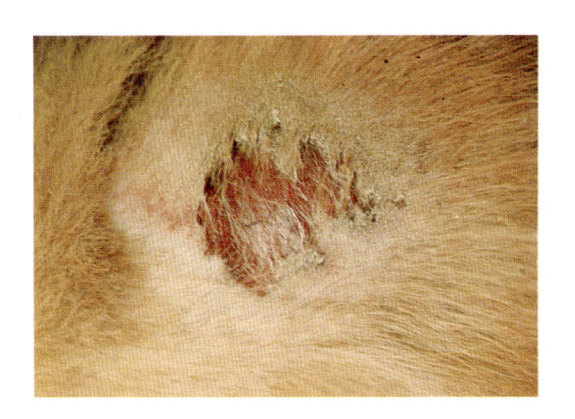

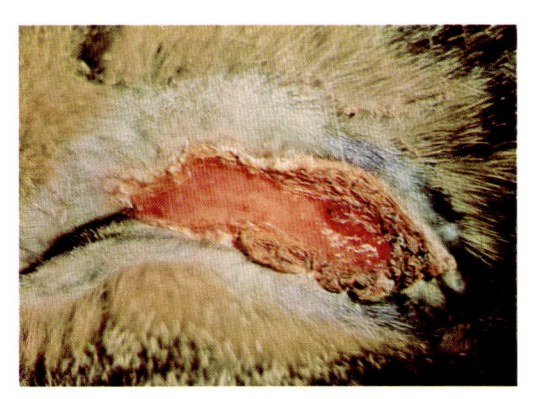

Fig. 195 A   Fig. 195 B

(Cat). A patch of necrotic skin and an extensive deep ulcer resulting from prolonged contact with heating pads which were used postoperatively for hypothermia.

CHAPTER 18

INTERTRIGO

An erythematous eruption of the skin produced by friction of adjacent parts.

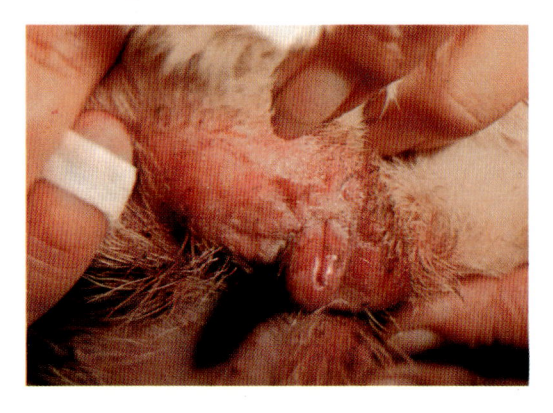

Fig. 196

Perivulvar intertrigo. The perivulvar folds have been pulled back to reveal an intertriginous dermatitis. This condition occurs frequently in obese, spayed females.

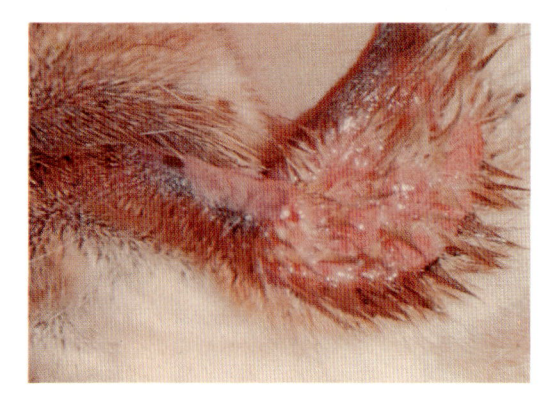

Fig. 197

Lip fold pyoderma. An ulcerated secondarily infected patch on the lower lip (in the area of the canine tooth).

CHAPTER
19

EOSINOPHILIC GRANULOMA

A chronic dermatosis occurring on the lips, oral mucosa and integument (particularly the abdomen) of cats of all ages and sexes. The cause of the disease is not known.

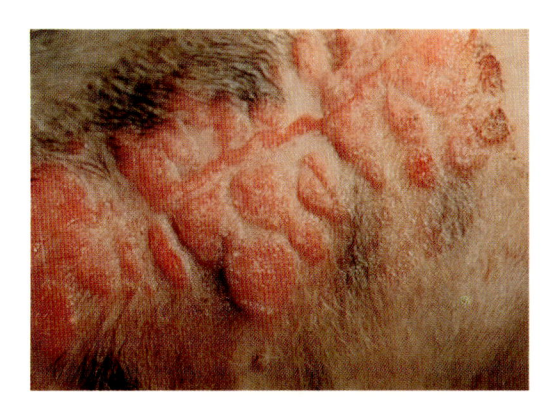

Fig. 198 A

Fig. 198 B

Erythematous ulcerative plaques on groin.

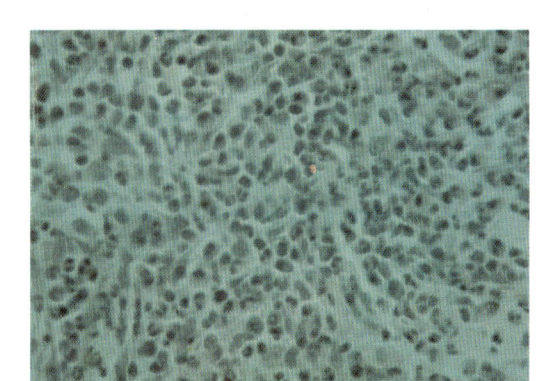

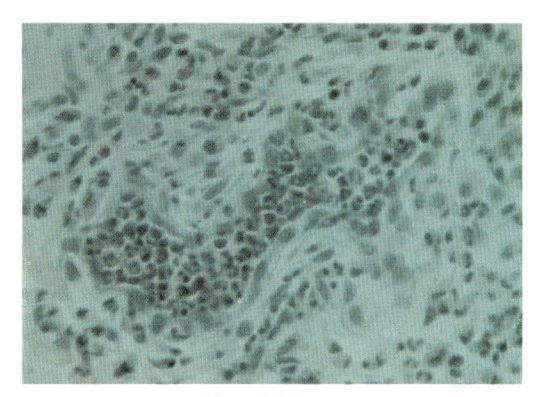

Fig. 199 A

Fig. 199 B

A dense inflammatory infiltrate of eosinophils and histiocytes is the predominant reaction in the dermis. The epidermis usually is absent and/or undergoing pseudo-epitheliomatous hyperplasia. H. & E., × 450.

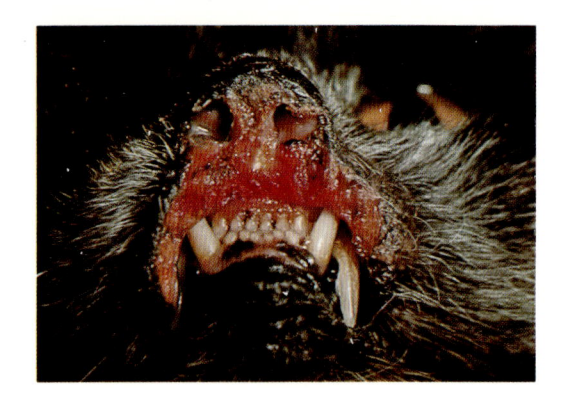

Fig. 200 A

Fig. 200 B

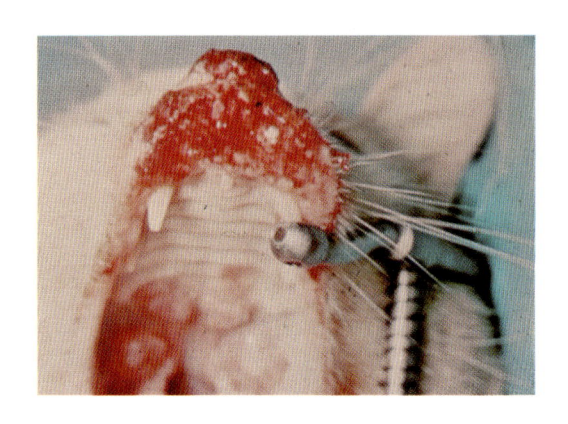

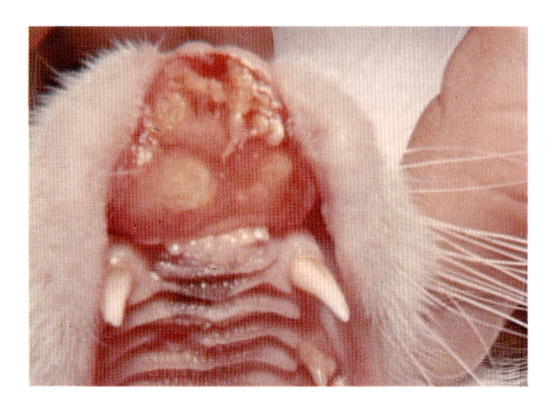

Fig. 200 C

Fig. 200 D

Oral lesions most often involve the upper lips and are ulcerative or erosive reactions.

CHAPTER
20

LINEAR GRANULOMA

A dermatosis of cats of unknown causation occurring on the upper aspects of the extremities and abdomen, and characterized by linear yellow or pinkish-yellow plaques. Lesions are bilateral and may or may not be pruritic or alopecic. The main histopathologic change is discrete areas of collagen degeneration and necrosis surrounded by a histiocytic and giant cell infiltrate.

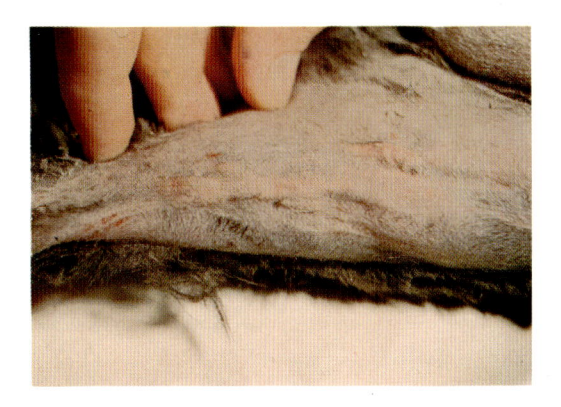

Fig. 201 A

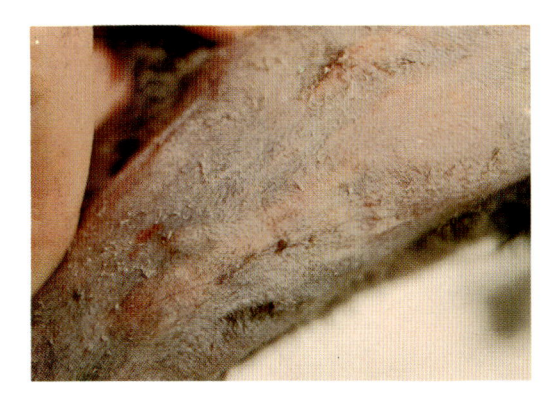

Fig. 201 B

Linear plaques on posterior aspects of thighs.

CHAPTER 21

ACNE

Comedones (blackheads) may occur on the lips and/or chin of cats of all ages and sexes. Lesions are non-pruritic and non-inflammatory. The cause of the dermatosis is not known though a hormonal aberration is suspect. In the dog, comedones usually occur on the scrotum, penile sheath and groin.

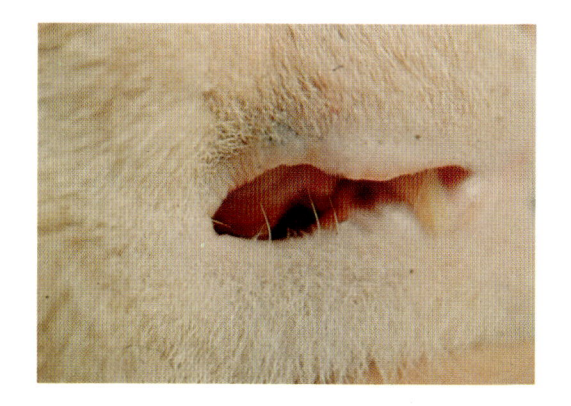

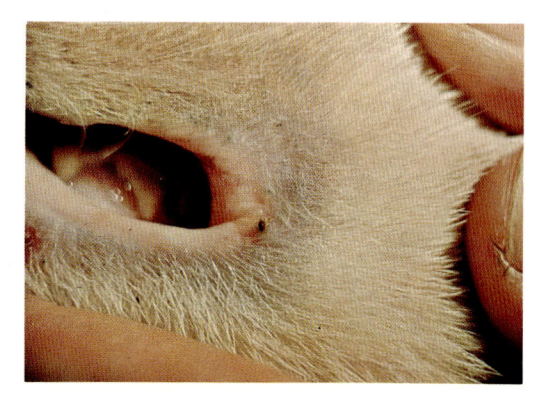

Fig. 202 A

Fig. 202 B

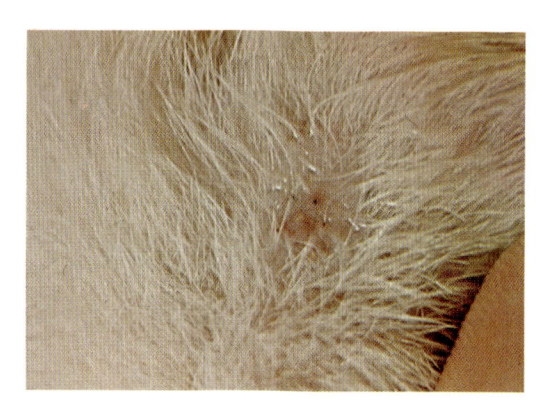

Fig. 202 C
(Cat). Comedones on lips and chin.

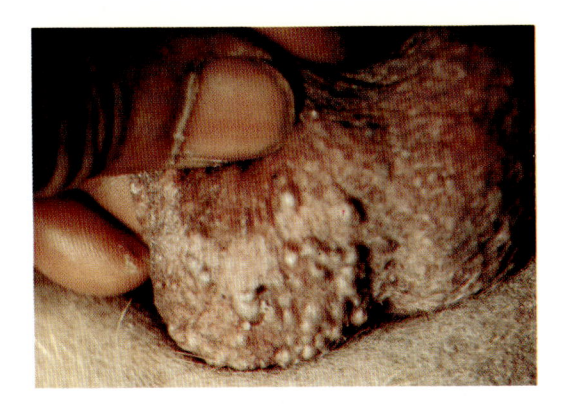

Fig. 203 A

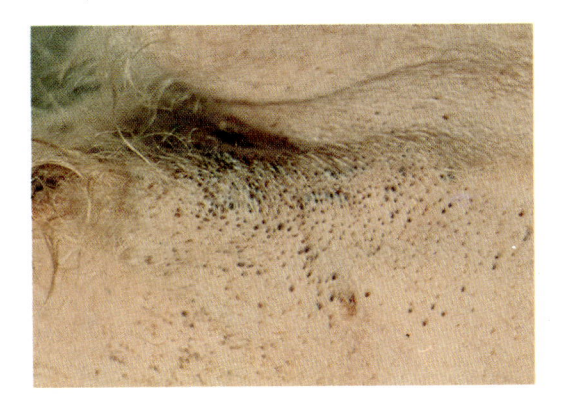

Fig. 203 B
Comedones on scrotum, penile sheath and groin.

CHAPTER 22

HORMONAL DERMATOSES

Hypothyroidism. The cutaneous manifestations associated with this thyroidal dysfunction are: bilaterally symmetrical alopecia (particularly on the dorsal aspects of the neck and lumbosacral back); a dull, lusterless pelage; and a rough scaling, (often) hyperpigmented skin.

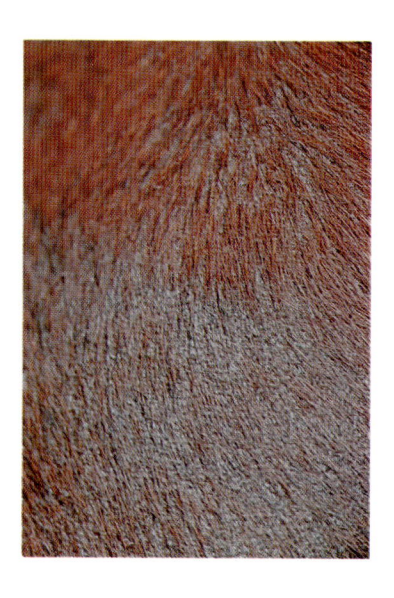

Fig. 204
Alopecia, hyperpigmentation and scaling on dorsal aspect of the neck.

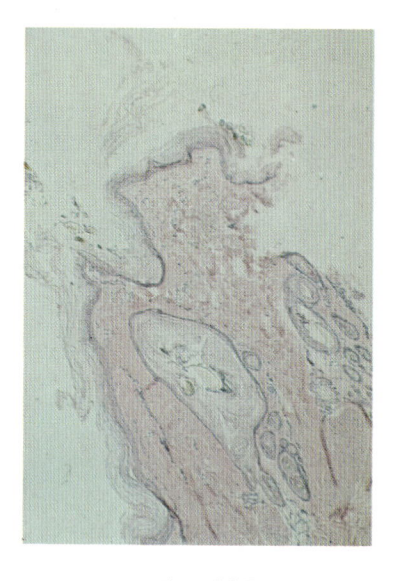

Fig. 205
Biopsy of lesion (Fig. 204). Note hyperkeratosis, thin-walled dilated follicle filled with keratotic material, and edema in upper part of dermis. H. & E., × 35.

Fig. 206

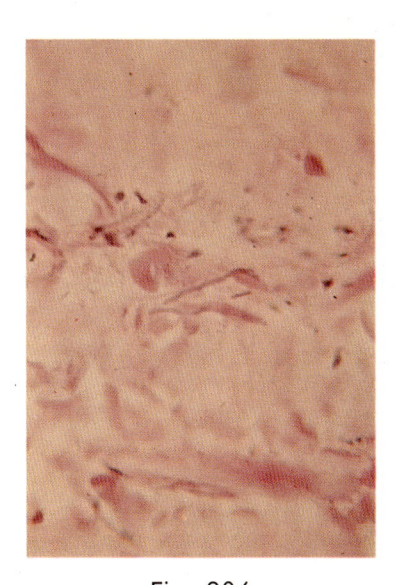

Biopsy of lesion (Fig. 204). Note swollen homogeneous collagen and basophilic strands in dermis. H. & E., × 450.

ACANTHOSIS NIGRICANS

This disease most often is related to a dysfunction of the pituitary thyroid axis (gonad or adrenal aberrations also may be causative). It occurs commonly in the Dachshund breed and is characterized by hyperpigmented lichenified patches or plaques on the axilla (initially), groin, ventral aspect of the neck and pinna. Seborrheic disorders commonly are associated.

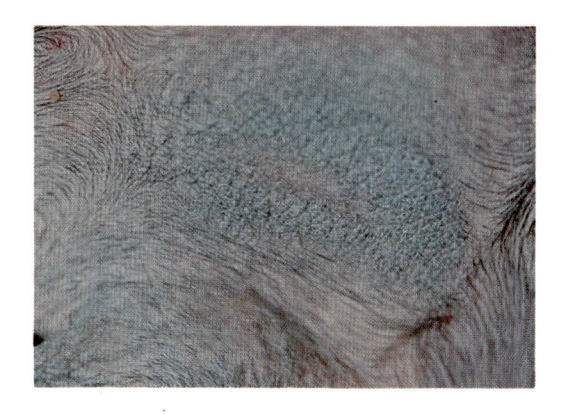

Fig. 207
An annular pigmented lichenified plaque on axilla.

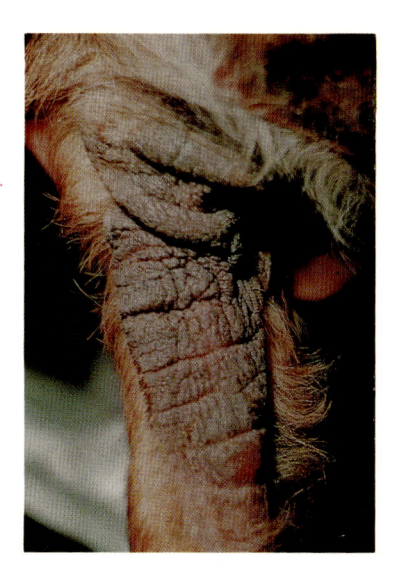

Fig. 208
Hyperpigmentation and lichenification on axilla and inner aspect of forearm.

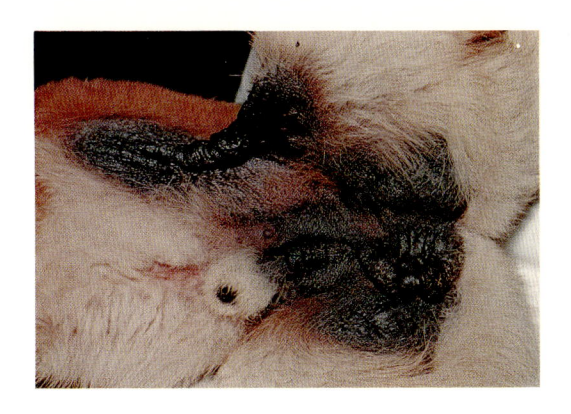

Fig. 209
Later involvement of groin (patient in Fig. 208).

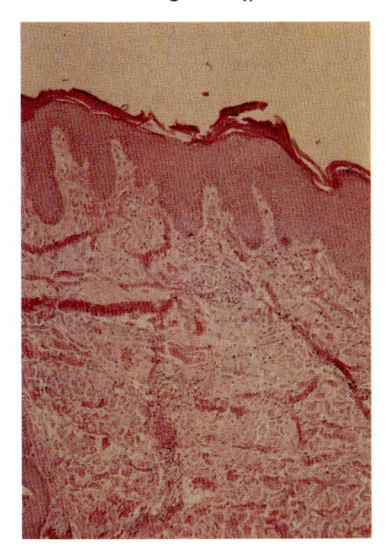

Fig. 210
Biopsy of lesion (Fig. 208). Note parakeratosis, acanthosis with ridging and a minimal sub-acute inflammatory infiltration in upper portion of the dermis. H. & E., × 100.

GONADAL-ADRENAL DYSFUNCTION

Aberrations of these organs are grouped together because they often are manifested by similar cutaneous lesions: alopecia, seborrheic disorders, hyperpigmentation, lichenification, sweating and occasionally marked pruritus. The areas of involvement also are similar: folds of the flank, groin and perineum (initially) with later involvement of the abdomen, axilla, neck and lower part of the back. As few specific clinico-pathology tests have not been developed for the diagnosis of hormonal disease in dogs and cats, the word dysfunction is used in most cases rather than specifying the specific hormonal problem.

TESTICULAR DYSFUNCTION

Sertoli Cell Tumor Syndrome. This estrogen producing tumor usually develops in a retained testicle and results in a feminizing syndrome. Cutaneous changes include: gynecomastia, generalized alopecia (the head and extremities usually are spared), scaling and lichenification on the abdomen.

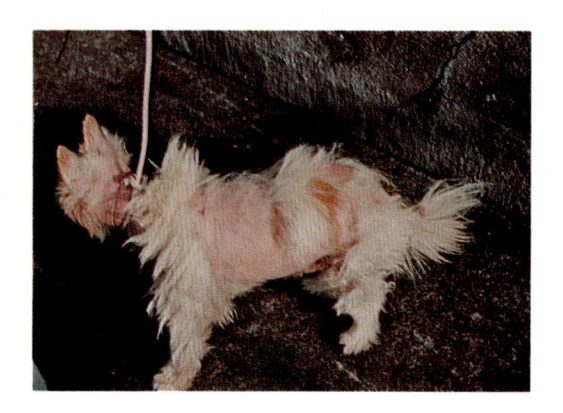

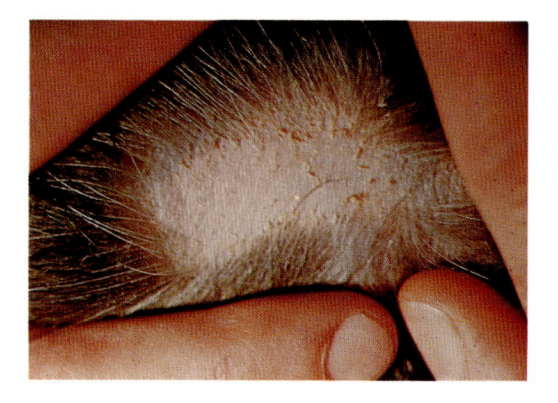

Fig. 211

Hairs of the trunk are in telogen and can be epilated with ease. The pattern of alopecia is conditioned by friction—in this case, the wearing of a harness produced the alopecia on the neck and chest.

Fig. 212

Hair has been epilated from the trunk. A smooth normal appearing skin surface (other than fine yellow scaling) is evident.

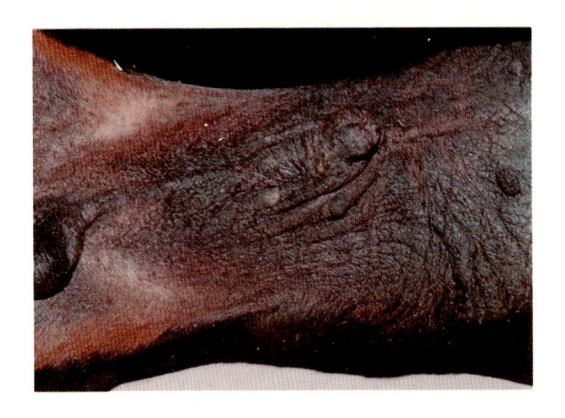

Fig. 213
Note lichenification, hyperpigmentation and gynecomastia.

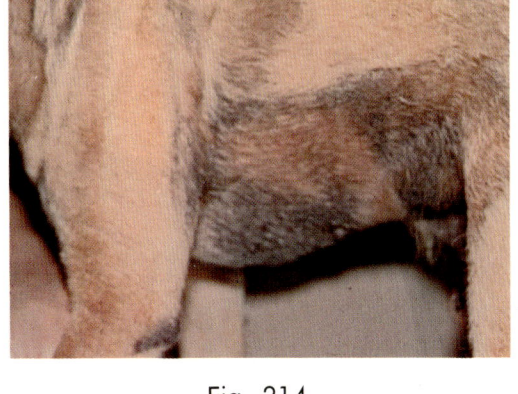

Fig. 214
Note hyperpigmentation and lichenification on abdomen (hair has been removed for visualization of lesion).

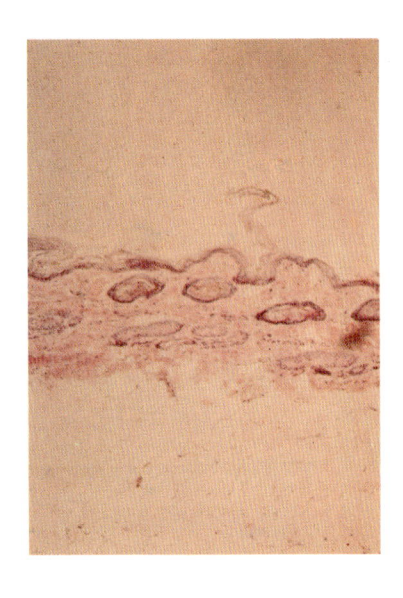

Fig. 215
Biopsy of alopecic patch (Fig. 211). Note marked atrophy of skin and dilated follicles filled with keratin. H. & E., ×35.

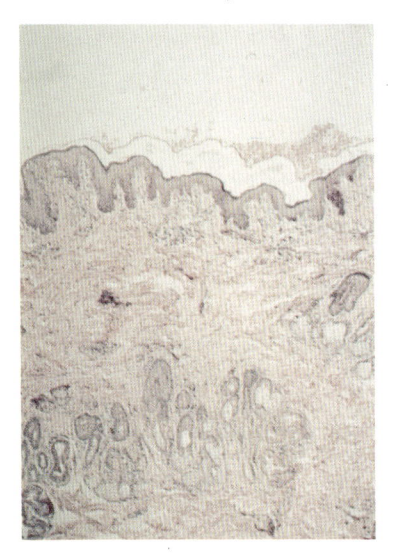

Fig. 216
Biopsy of lichenified patch (Fig. 213). Note acanthosis with ridging and minimal patchy chronic inflammatory infiltrate in upper portion of dermis. H. & E., ×35.

HYPOANDROGENISM

A testicular dysfunction corrected by testosterone replacement therapy; and characterized by aspermatogenesis, hyperpigmentation and lichenification on the groin and perineum (initially and later the axilla), seborrheic disorders and a ceruminous otitis externa.

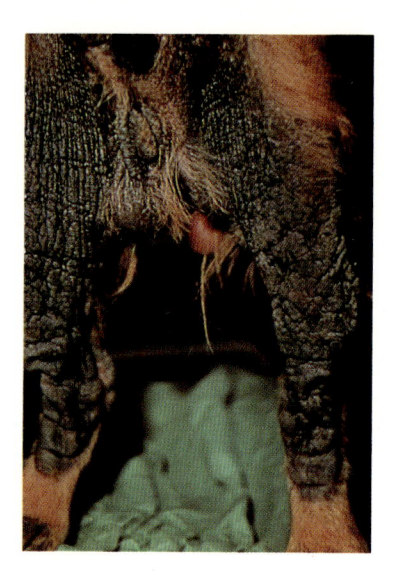

Fig. 217
Note hyperpigmentation and lichenification on groin.

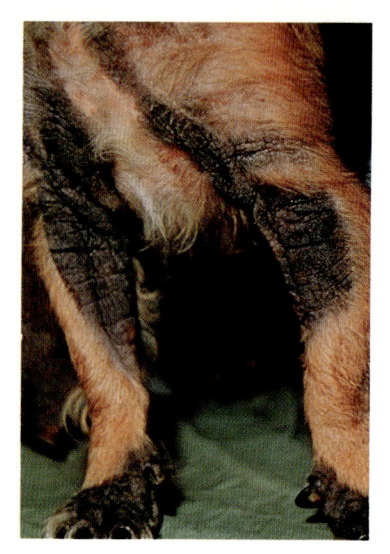

Fig. 218
Similar lesions on axillae and digits.

OVARIAN DYSFUNCTION

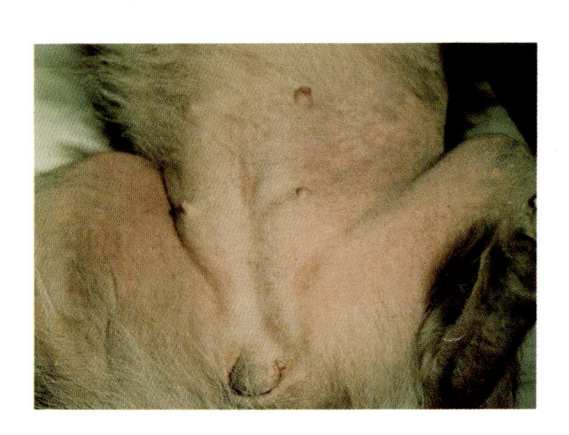

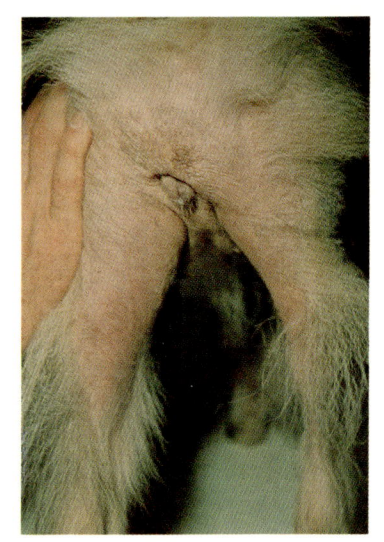

Fig. 219 A   Fig. 219 B

Alopecia on groin and perineal region associated with pseudocyesis (corrected by spaying).

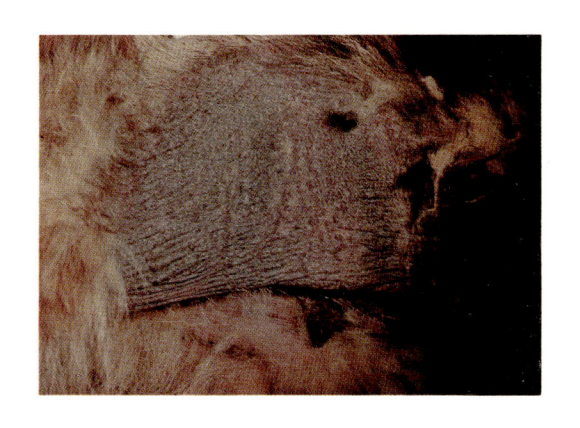

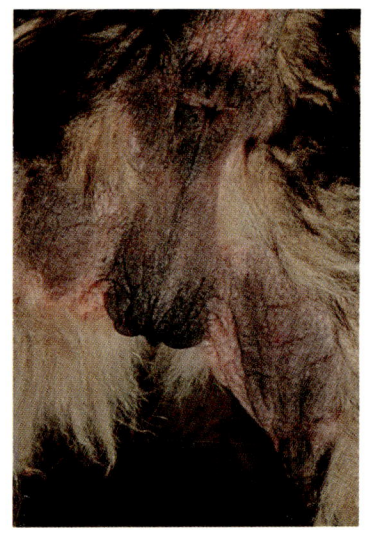

Fig. 220 A   Fig. 220 B

Alopecia, lichenification and hyperpigmentation on perineum and groin associated with anestrus and pseudocyesis.

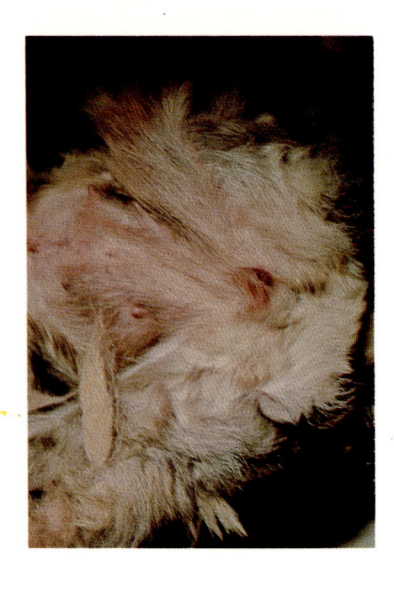

Fig. 221
Resolution of skin changes (patient in Fig. 220) one month following spay.

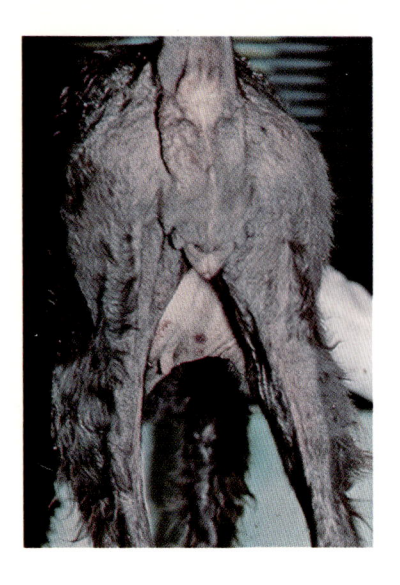

Fig. 222
Alopecia and hyperpigmentation on perineum associated with cystic ovaries.

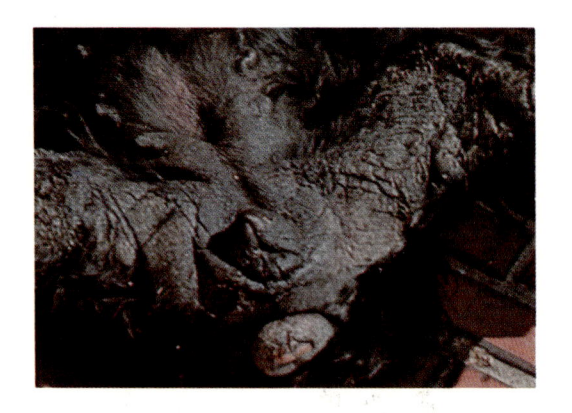

Fig. 223
Alopecia, hyperpigmentation and lichenification on perineum and groin associated with anestrus (corrected by spaying).

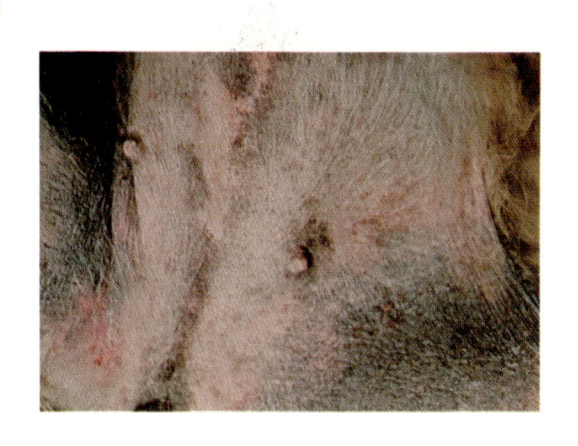

Fig. 224 A 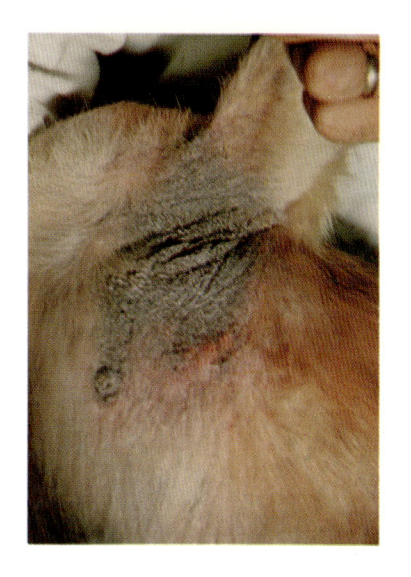   Fig. 224 B

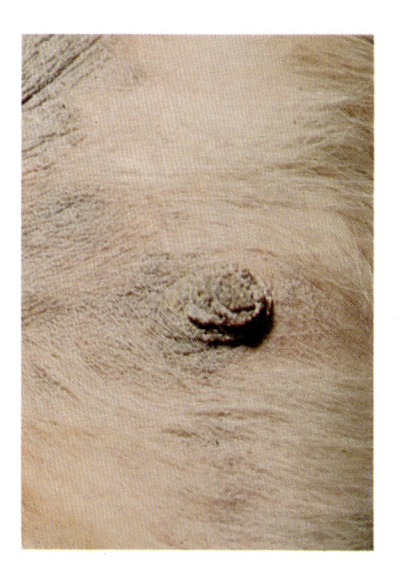

Fig. 224 C 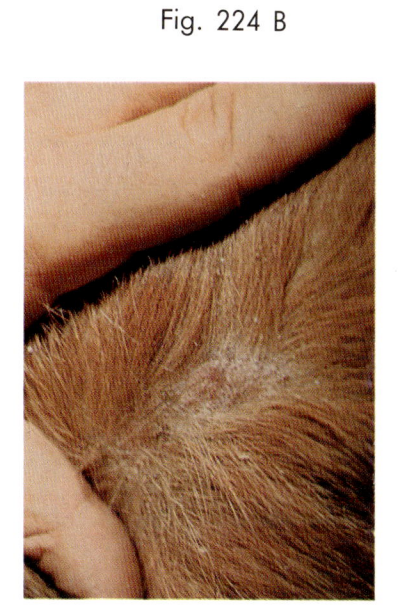   Fig. 224 D

Lichenification, hyperpigmentation and peripheral erythema on groin and axilla; crusting of nipple; and seborrhea (trunk) associated with pseudocyesis (corrected by spaying).

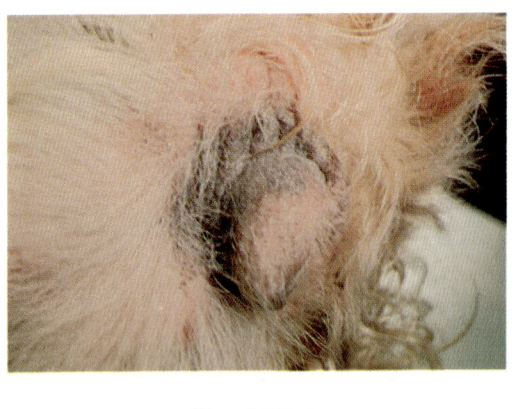

Fig. 225 A

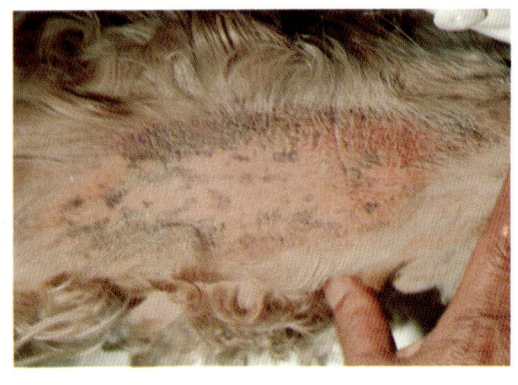

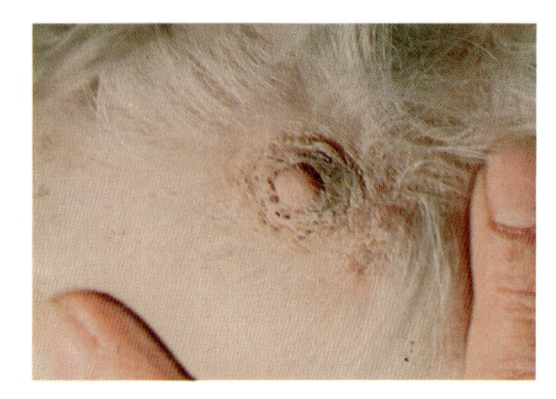

Fig. 225 B

Fig. 225 C

Fig. 225 D

Hyperpigmentation, lichenification and alopecia on vulva, fold of the flanks and ventral aspect of the neck; and enlargement and crusting of nipple associated with anestrus and pseudocyesis.

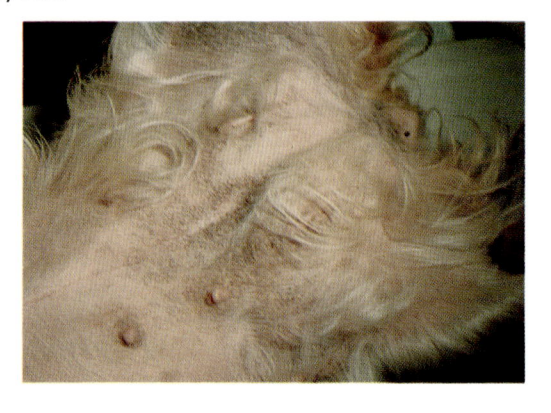

Fig. 226

Note regrowth of hair and resolution of lichenified lesions one month following spay (patient in Fig. 225 A-D). Milk is still present in breasts.

CHANGES OCCURRING WITH CASTRATION

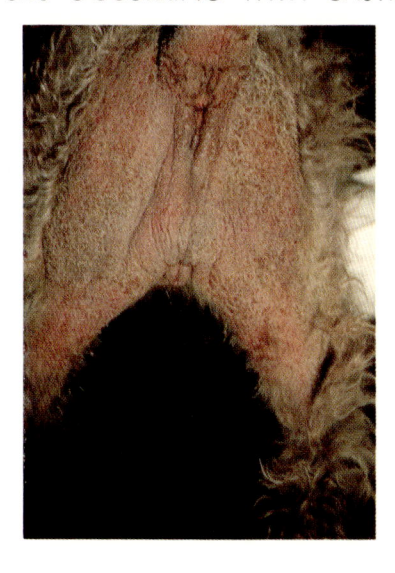

Fig. 227

Alopecia, scaling and erythema on perineum. Animal was spayed at six months of age and dermatosis developed during the seventh year of life. Condition corrected by estrogen replacement therapy.

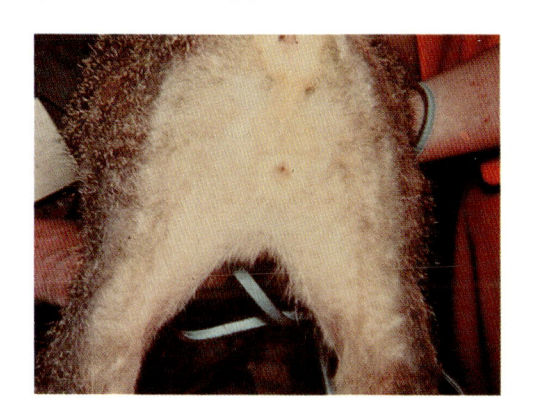

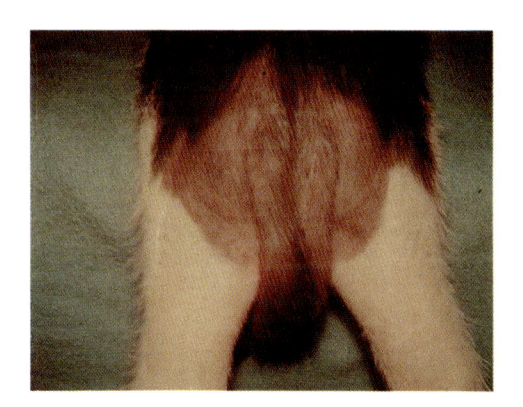

Fig. 228 A   Fig. 228 B

(Cat). Alopecia on perineum developing two years after castration. Corrected with testosterone replacement therapy.

ADRENAL DYSFUNCTION

Cushing's Disease. The cutaneous changes resulting from an overproduction of 17 hydroxycorticosteroids are: thinning and wrinkling of the skin, alopecia, an erythematous macular and papular eruption, hyperpigmented macules, subcutaneous plaques and calcinosis cutis.

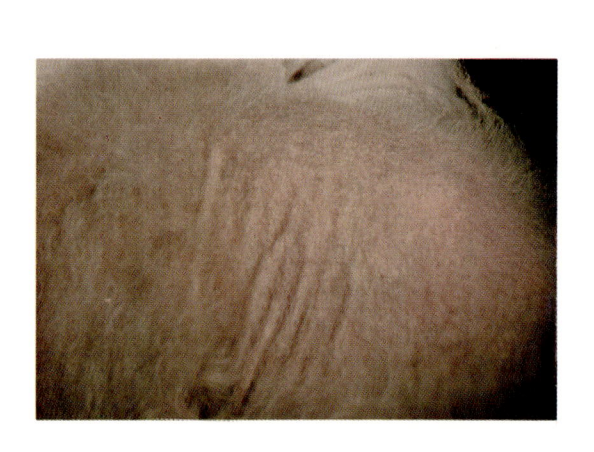

Fig. 229 A 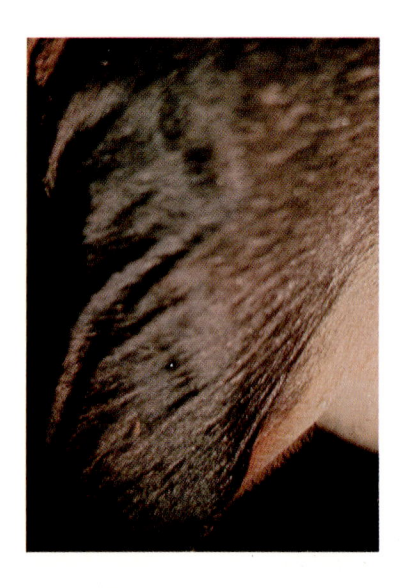   Fig. 229 B

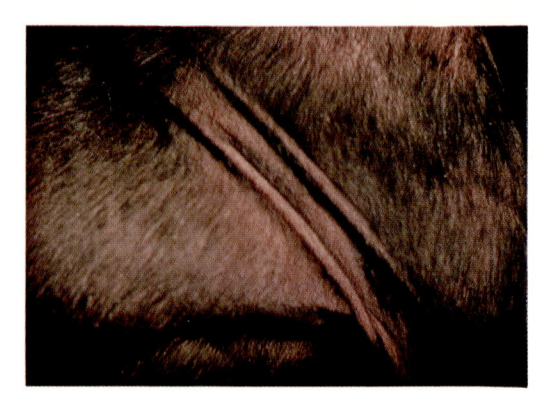

Fig. 229 C
The skin when picked up into folds remains wrinkled rather than snapping back into normal position.

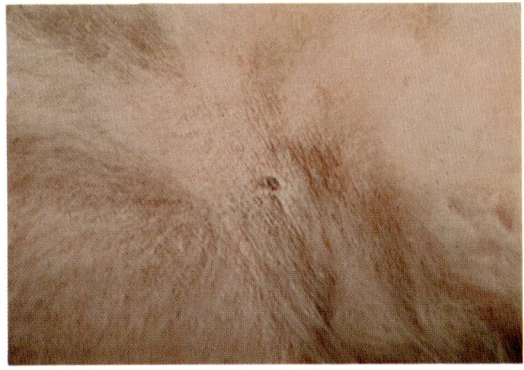

Fig. 230

A hyperpigmented macule on lateral aspect of the chest. Lesion is the result of hemorrhage in upper one-half of the dermis. (See Fig. 237).

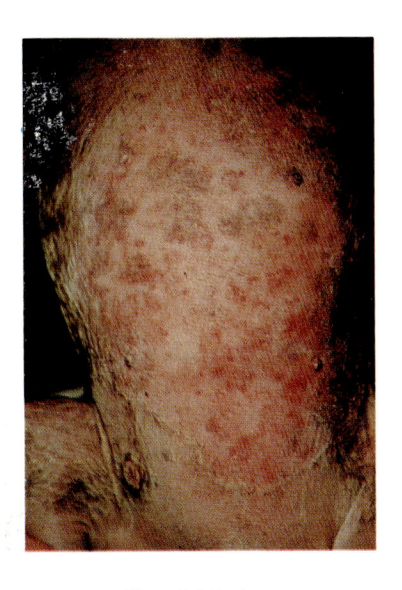

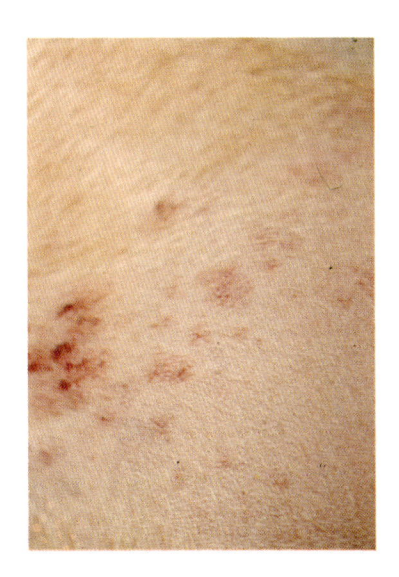

Fig. 231 A   Fig. 231 B

An erythematous macular and papular eruption on chest and lateral aspect of the neck.

101

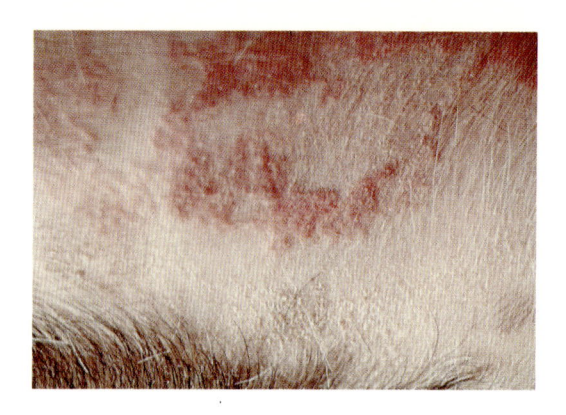

Fig. 232
Calcinosis cutis. Erythematous plaques on groin.

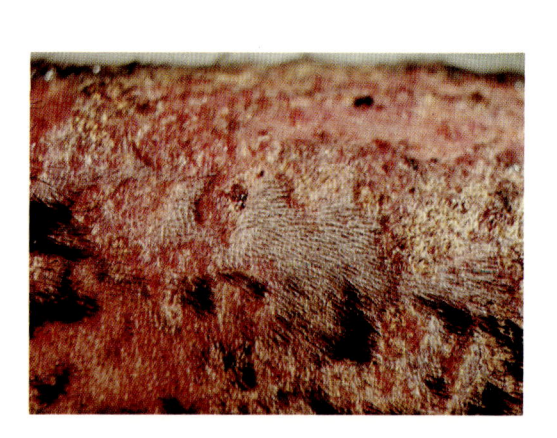

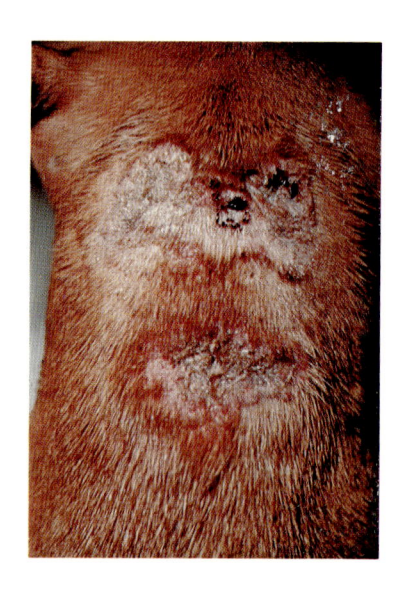

Fig. 233 A   Fig. 233 B
Calcinosis cutis. Erythematous plaques on neck.

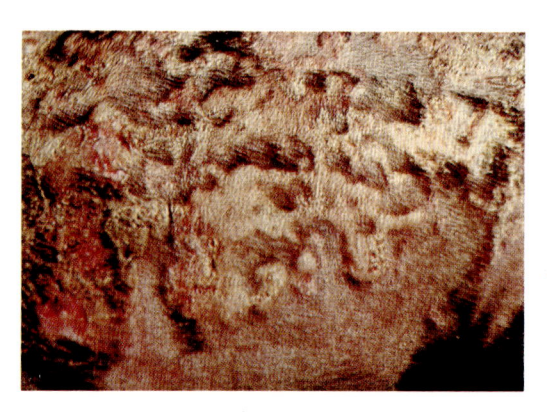

Fig. 234
Calcinosis cutis. A yellow crust overlays erythematous plaques—resembling a pyoderma.

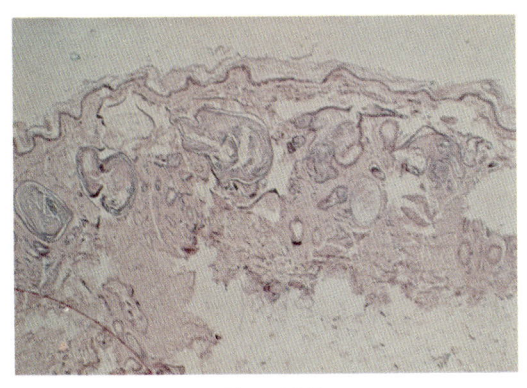

Fig. 235
Biopsy of lesion (Fig. 229 A). Note marked atrophy of skin, hyperkeratosis and distended follicles filled with keratin. H. & E., ×35.

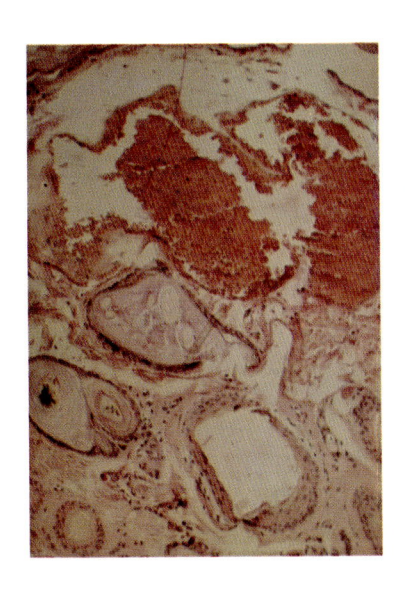

Fig. 236
Biopsy of lesion (Fig. 229 A). Note edematous appearance of dermis and follicular orifices filled with keratin. H. & E., ×100.

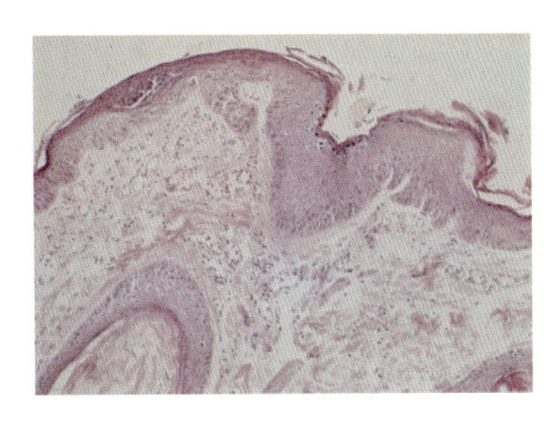

Fig. 237
Biopsy of lesion (Fig. 230). Note hemorrhage in the upper portion of the dermis. H. & E., ×100.

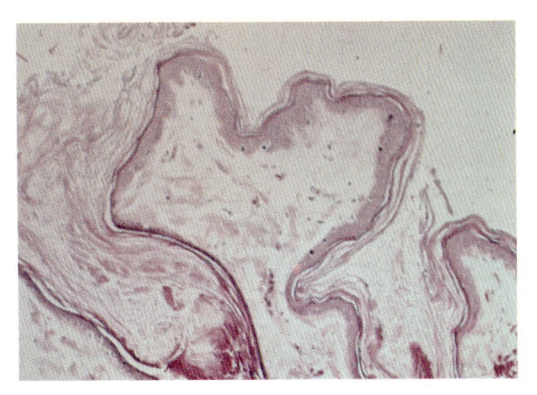

Fig. 238
Biopsy of lesion (Fig. 231 B). The epidermis is parakeratotic and acanthotic (with ridging). In the upper part of the dermis, vascular dilatation, edema and an inflammatory infiltration are present. H. & E., ×100.

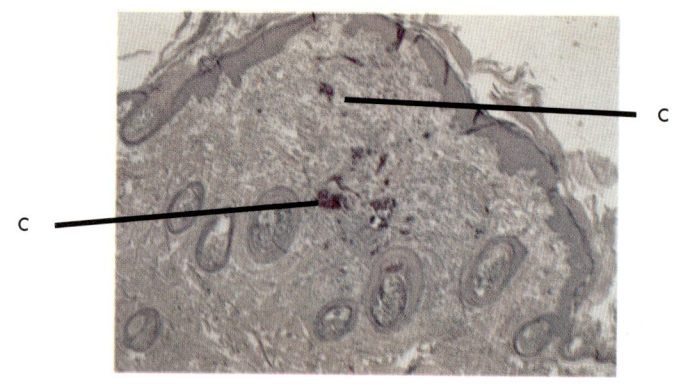

Fig. 239

Biopsy of lesion (Fig. 234). The epidermis is hyperkeratotic and acanthotic. Calcification (c) and a chronic inflammatory infiltrate are present in the upper one-half of the dermis. H. & E., ×100.

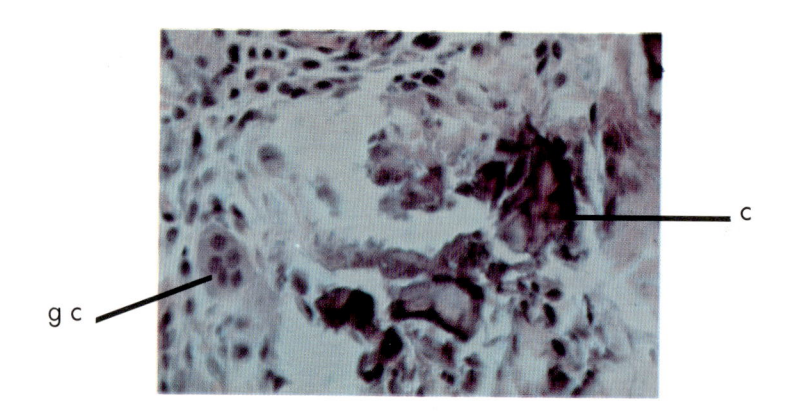

Fig. 240

Biopsy of lesion (Fig. 234). Note calcification (c) and giant cell (g c). H. & E., ×400.

CUTANEOUS LESION ASSOCIATED WITH INCREASED 17-KETOSTEROID OUTPUT

In the dog, the testicles, ovaries and adrenals produce 17-ketosteroids. Associated with increased production of the hormone are significant skin changes: alopecia, lichenification and hyperpigmentation on the abdomen and perineum, seborrheic disorders, alopecia on lower part of the back, hyperhidrosis, comedones and occassionally marked pruritus. Removal of the abnormally functioning gonads or adrenal is curative in approximately 50 per cent of the cases. As the pituitary drives the above mentioned organs, the origin of the pathology may be at this higher level with secondary involvement of the gonads or adrenals.

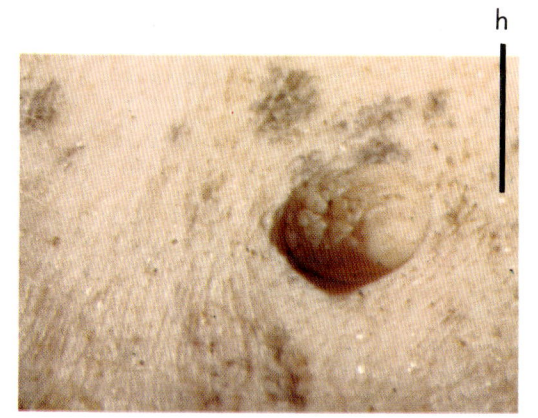

Fig. 241 A

Fig 241 B

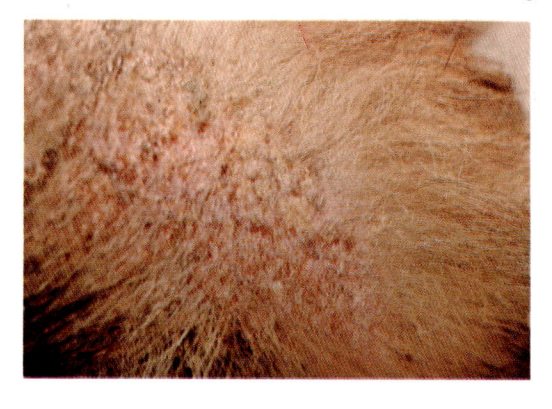

Fig. 241 C

Note hyperhidrosis (h) on abdomen and fold of flank, enlarged nipple, and alopecia and seborrheic dermatitis on median aspect of the back (24-hour urine 17-ketosteroids— 3.7 mg.).

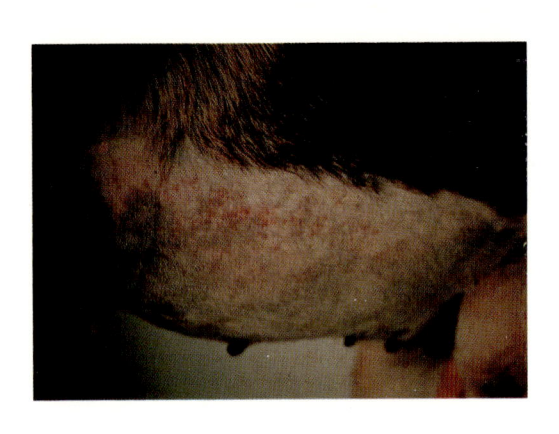

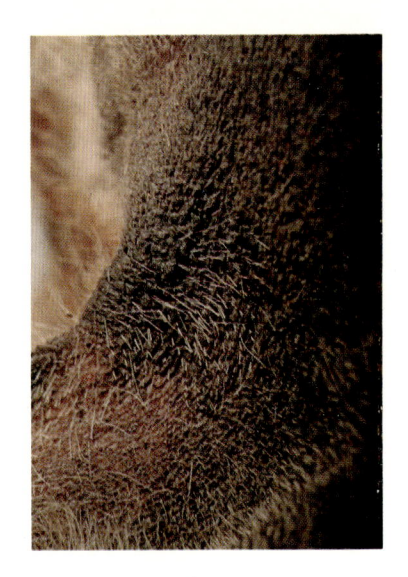

Fig. 242 A

Fig. 242 B

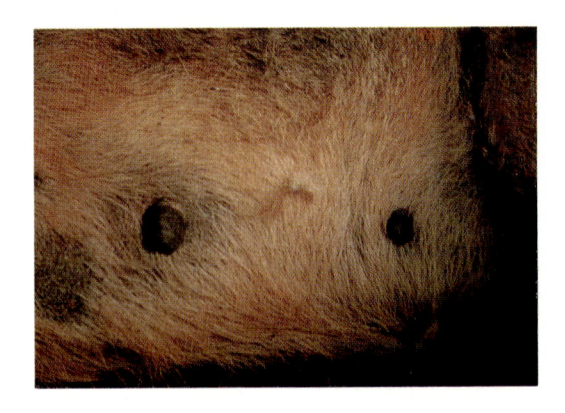

Fig. 242 C
Hair has been removed from abdomen in order to visualize lesions. Note hyperpigmentation and peripheral erythematous macular eruption on abdomen, axillary lichenification and enlarged pigmented nipples (hyperhidrosis present but not discernible in picture). Dog had fibrotic and cystic ovaries (24-hour urine 17-ketosteroid—3.1 mg.).

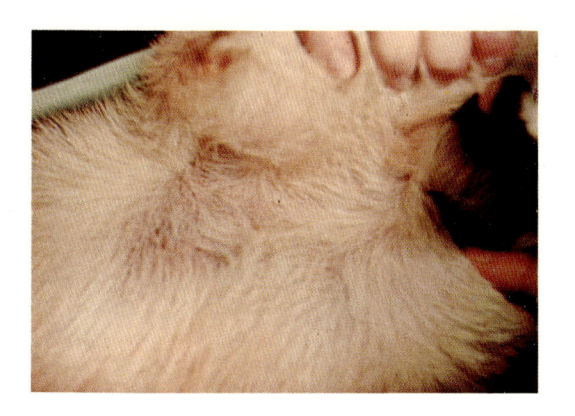

Fig. 243 A 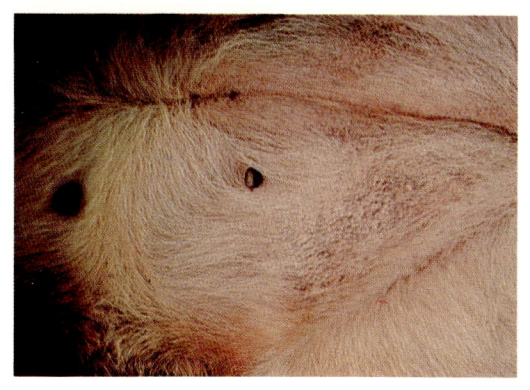   Fig. 243 B

One month following spaying, lesions are resolving (patient, Figs. 242 A, B, C).

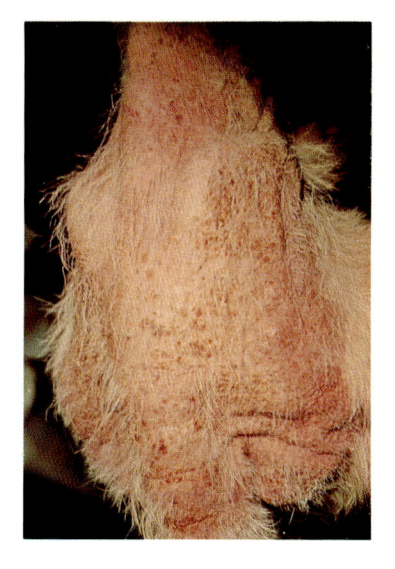

Fig. 244 A 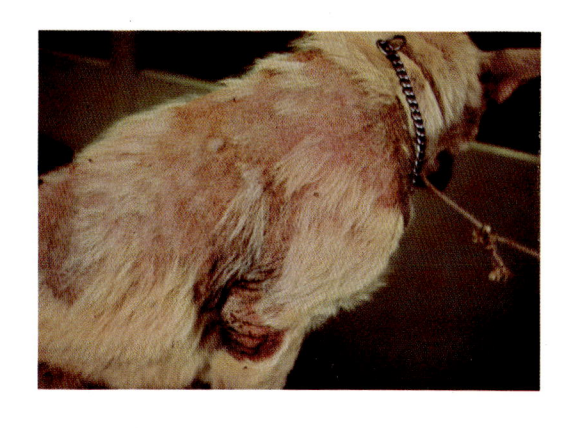   Fig. 244 B

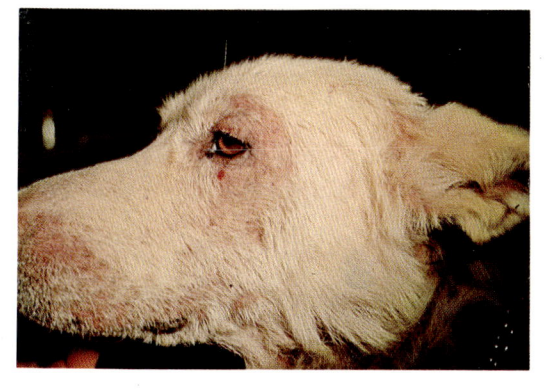

Fig. 244 C 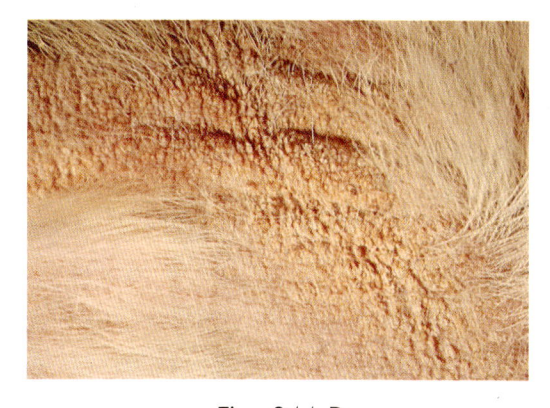   Fig. 244 D

Alopecia and a seborrheic dermatitis are present on abdomen, medial aspect of the back, scapular and neck areas, periocular and pre-auricular regions. Dog had a Sertoli cell tumor (24-hour urine values for estrogen was less than 12 mouse units and for 17-ketosteroids, 2.7 mg.).

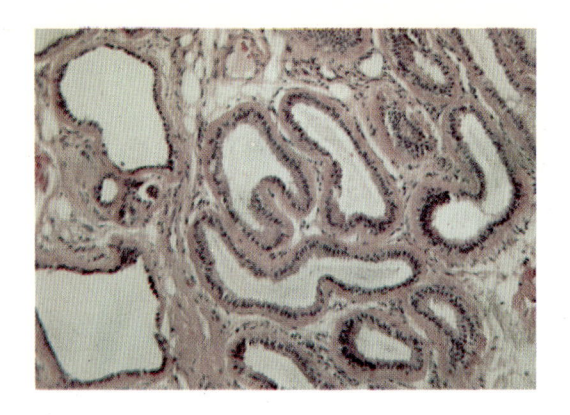

Fig. 245

Biopsy of lesion (Fig. 244 B). Apocrine structures are filled with their secretions and columnar epithelium is intact. H. & E., ×100.

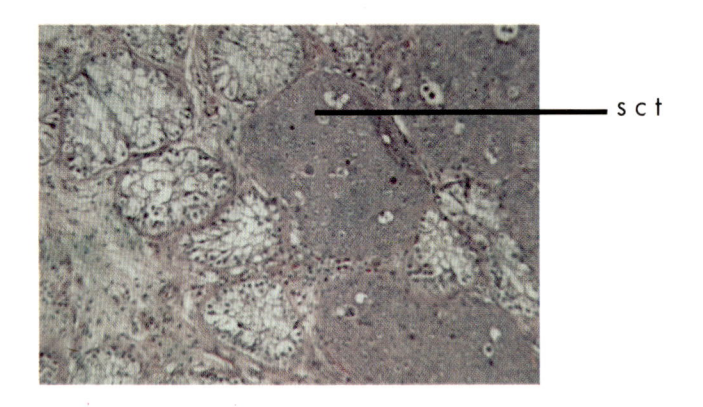

Fig. 246

Biopsy of testicle from patient (Fig. 244 A-D). Note Sertoli cell tumor (s c t). H. & E., ×100.

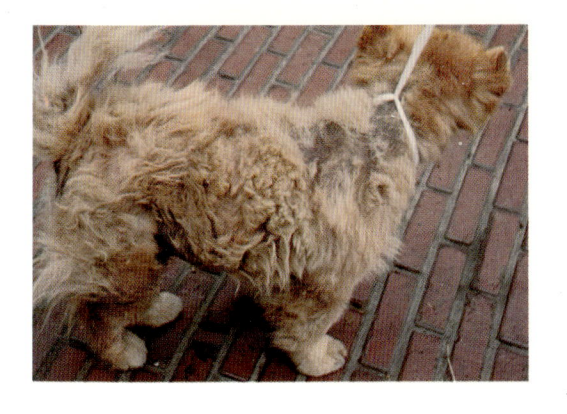

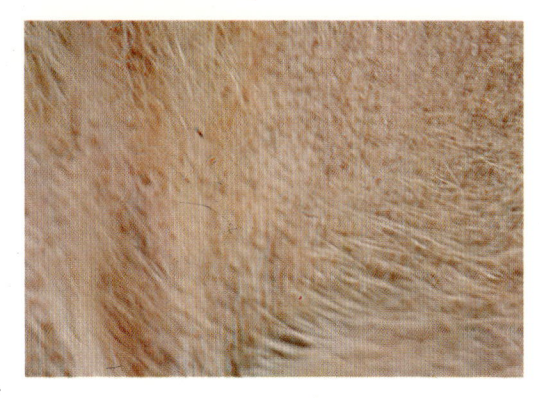

Fig. 247 A					Fig. 247 B

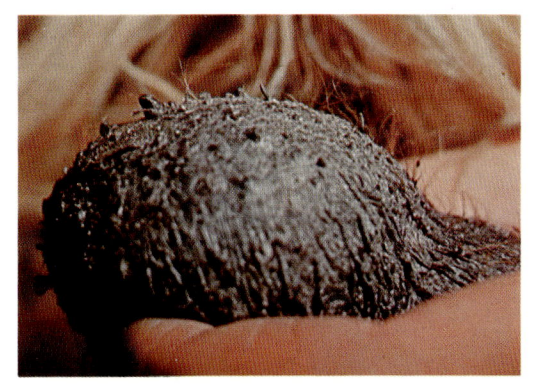

Fig. 247 C

Note dull hair coat, alopecia and hyperpigmentation on dorso-lateral aspect of the neck and shoulder region, hyperhidrosis (axilla) and scrotal comedones. Dog had an adrenal tumor (24-hour urine value for 17-ketosteroids, 4.3 mg.).

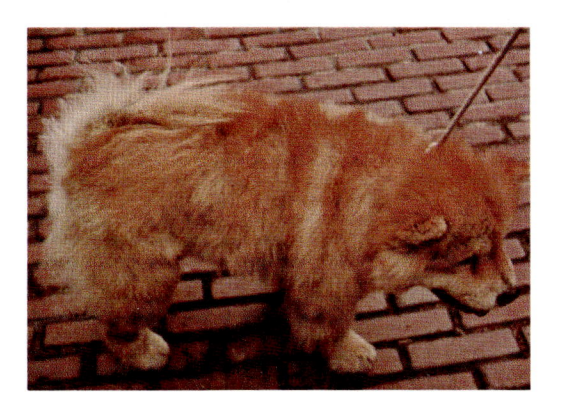

Fig. 248

Patient (Fig. 247) one month following adrenalectomy. Note regrowth of hair.

INDEX

Acanthosis, 24, 34, 91
Acanthosis nigricans, 90
Acne, 86 (also see, comedo)
Acral-pruritic nodules, 79
Adrenal dysfunction, 100
Allergic contact dermatitis, 31
Allergic dermatoses, 28
Alopecia, 16, 32, 55, 56, 59, 63, 66, 70, 73, 74, 88, 93, 95, 96, 98, 99, 105, 107, 109
Anagen, 20
Anagen cat hair, 22
Anagen dog hair, 21
Anestrus, 95, 96, 98
Aspermatogenesis, 94
Atopy, 30

Bacterial infection, 39 (also see, pyoderma)
Bacterial paronychia, 46
Basic reaction of skin, 11-27
Blackheads, 86 (also see, comedo)
Blastomycosis, North American, 51, 52
Blister, 12
Bulla, 12, 25

C. albicans, 68
C. parasitivorax, 61
Calcinosis cutis, 100, 102
Callus, 77
Callus, infected, 49
Castration, changes occurring, 99
Cat, skin of, 21
Cellulitis, 77
Cheyletiella parasitivorax dermatitis, 61, 62
Comedo, 15
Comedones, 86, 87, 105, 109
Contact dermatitis, 31
Crusting, 53, 57, 59, 63, 70, 73, 97
Crusts, 17
Cushing's disease, 100

Definitions, 11-27
Demodectic mange, 50, 55
Demodectic mite, 57, 58
Depigmentation, 15, 33
Depigmentation of nares, 32
Dermatitis, acute, 26
Dermatitis, Cheyletiella parasitivorax, 61, 62
Dermatitis, chronic, 27
Dermatitis, contact, 31
Dermatitis, rhabditic, 59
Dermatitis, solar, 32
Dermatomycosis, 64

Dermatophytes, 64
Dermatoses, allergic, 28
Dermatoses, hormonal, 88

Ear mite infestation, 47
Eczematoid dermatitis, 50
Eosinophilic granuloma, 83
Epidermis, 18
Erythema, 11, 33, 59, 99
Erythema, interdigital, 75
Erythema, peripheral, 97
Erythematous nodules, 41
Erythematous papules, 53
Estrogen replacement therapy, 99
Exudation, 12

Facial keratosis, 73
Flea bites, 36, 37, 38
Fleas, 49
Follicular destruction, 26
Follicular keratosis, 73
Folliculitis, 40
Furuncle, biopsy, 42
Furuncular lesions, 56
Furunculosis, 41, 50, 57
Furunculosis, interdigital, 42
Furunculosis, labial, 42

Gonadal-adrenal dysfunction, 92
Granuloma, eosinophilic, 83
Granuloma, linear, 85
Gynecomastia, 92, 93

Hair follicle, 20
Hard pad disease, 51
Hives, 28
Hidradenitis suppurativa, 44
Histology, 18-23
Histopathologic reactions, 23-27
Hormonal dermatoses, 88
Hyperhidrosis, 105, 106, 109
Hyperkeratosis, 103
Hyperpigmentation, 57, 59, 88, 92, 93, 95, 98, 105, 109
Hyperplasia of granular cell layer, 24
Hyperplasia, pseudoepitheliomatous, 83
Hyphae, 67
Hypoandrogenism, 94
Hypothyroidism, 23, 88

Impetigo, 39
Intertrigo, 82
Intoxication, thallium, 74

Juvenile pyoderma, 45

Keratosis, 73
Keratosis, facial, 73
Keratosis, follicular, 73

Leptospirosis, 51
Lichenification, 15, 92, 93, 95, 97, 98, 105
Lichenification, axillary, 106
Linear granuloma, 85
Liquefaction degeneration, 24

M. canis, 64, 65, 66, 67
M. gypsum, 64, 65
Macules, 11
Macules, hyperpigmentated, 100, 101
Mange, demodectic, 50, 55
Mange, notoedric, 63
Mange, sarcoptic, 53
Melanin production, 27
Moniliasis, 68

N. cati, 63
Nail bed, infection of, 46
Necrosis, 16
Necrotizing pyoderma, 45
Nematode, 59
Nocardiosis, 52
Nodules, acral-pruritic, 79
Notoedric mange, 63

Otitis externa, 94
Ovarian dysfunction, 95

Pad of normal dog, 19
Papule, 13, 73
Parakeratosis, 23, 76, 91
Paronychia, bacterial, 46
Patches, erythematous, 72
Perivulvar intertrigo, 82
Pigmentation, 94
Plaque, 13
Plaque, erythematous, 43, 68, 72, 78, 102
Plaque, lichenified, 90
Plaque, pigmented, 78
Plaque, ulcerated, 43
Plaques, furuncular, 56
Plaques, linear, 85
Plaques, moist, 44
Plaques, subcutaneous, 100
Pollinosis, 30
Pruritus, 28, 30, 92, 105
Pseudoepitheliomatous hyperplasia, 83
Pseudocyesis, 95, 98
Pustule, 13
Pustule, biopsy of, 40
Pustule, spongiform, 25, 76

Pyoderma, 39, 102
Pyoderma, juvenile, 45
Pyoderma, lip fold, 82
Pyoderma, necrotizing, 45
Pyoderma, secondary, 46
Pyoderma, staphylococcal, 44

R. strongyloides, 59, 60
Ragweed, reactions to, 30
Reticular degeneration, 25
Rhabditic dermatitis, 59
Ringworm, 26
Rodenticide, 74

Sarcoptic mites, 54
Scabies, 53
Scales, 17
Scaling, 70, 73, 88, 99
Scratch test, 30
Seborrhea, 70, 97
Seborrhea oleosa, 71
Seborrheic dermatitis, 72, 107
Seborrheic disorders, 90, 105
Secondary pyoderma, 46
Sertoli cell tumor, 107, 108
Sertoli cell tumor syndrome, 92
17-hydroxycorticosteroid, 100
17-ketosteroid output, 105
Skin of normal cat, 22
Skin of normal dog, 18, 19, 22, 23
Slough, 81
Solar dermatitis, 32
Spongiform pustule, 25, 76
Spores, 67
Staphylococcal organisms, 39
Syndrome, feminizing, 92

T. mentagrophytes, 65
Telogen, 20
Telogen cat hair, 22
Testicular dysfunction, 92, 94
Testosterone replacement therapy, 94, 99
Thallium intoxication, 23, 74
Tick bite, 34, 35
Trauma, self-inflicted, 47
Tumor, 13

Ulcer, 18
Ulcer, punched-out, 52
Ulceration, 75
Ulcerative dermatitis, 68
Urticaria, 25, 28

Viral infection, distemper-like, 51
Vitiligo, 15

Warts, canine, 24
Wheal, 14, 28